Confidence is Queen

Confidence is an inside job

Jen Sugermeyer

This book is dedicated to all the Queens.

Here are a few that have inspired me:

Julia Haart- for Pivoting

Ellen DeGeneres- for Pioneering

Oprah Winfrey- for Pushing

Sarah Blakely- for Paving

Brene' Brown- for Perceiving

Maya Angelou- for Poeticizing

Jennifer Vaughan- Prevailing

Danny Lee Cabrera- for Proving

Sakshi Tulsian- for Pursuing

Donna Sugermeyer- for Praising

Katie Pasquarella- for Promoting

Olive Pasquarella- for Playing

Jen Sugermeyer- for Persisting

CONTENTS

ACKNOWLEDGMENTS

I want to thank the amazing people that have inspired me and helped me to learn and grow.

I'd like to thank my parents, Bob & Donna Sugermeyer, for their support in getting through this book. And, for putting up with all my pivots throughout life!

I'd like to thank David Bayer for his teachings and continual quest for knowledge to make the world better.

John Christoph for help with the amazing cover. Nick Mallouf for the beautiful headshot.

For all of those that have supported me along my own journey, I appreciate you.

It takes a village.
It takes acts of kindness.
It takes patience.
It takes practice.
It takes confidence.

Whoever you are- I see you. You are never alone. You were made uniquely and perfectly you.

I love you.

Chapter 1: You Have it Inside of You

When I talk to individuals or companies about their goals they're always asking *how*. How to make more revenue. How to get into a relationship. How to find happiness. How to build a business. How to get out of suffering. How to get rid of toxicity. How to get healthy. How to lose weight.

Goal -> How to solve

By this point, they've likely tried at least one solution:

- Getting out in front of more ideal clients
- Showing up at more networking events
- Changing jobs
- Finding a new company to invest in
- Finding a new group of friends
- Changing diet or exercising more

Something's missing. They're still not where they want to be. What I'd like to offer is a *way* for you achieve everything you want in life. Whatever you're looking to accomplish, if you grasp this *way* of being then you'll find that everything is possible. The *way* is the fuel to get to the *how*. It's like the motor in a car. You need it to get to where you're going, otherwise you just have the tin shell.

It's a way to experience life more powerfully. A way to feel comfortable trying new things and saying YES more to new opportunities. A way to look in the mirror and see the support you need to get through everything. A way to show up in life authentically and unapologetically. A way to fuel your passion and your purpose.

Once you understand the way, then your options for how become limitless.

I have a little secret to share with you.

Everything you need is already inside of you: the answers, the strength, the how. The way to it is to tap into your confidence.

Regardless of every preconceived notion you may have, confidence is an inside job. Yes, you can put on an outfit you feel good in and dial up that confidence. You can pull your shoulders back and walk with intention. You can get your hair done and put on heels that make you feel like a million bucks. That will only get you so

8

far. The inside is where the magic happens and is that motor that will keep you in forward motion. Your actions, your demeanor, the way you show up is a direct reflection of what is happening on the inside. Everything boils down to confidence.

Takes confidence to love yourself, to take control of your life, to start a new business, to jump into a relationship, to start a family, to ask for that raise, to change jobs, to hang out by yourself, to show up every day and do the dang thing! Confidence is constantly coming into play in your life if you realize it or not. Confidence is the way to get everything you can dream out of this life.

I want this book to be more than just another motivational, rah-rah kind of book. I want this to transform the way you show up in your everyday life. I want you to walk away and know how to take control of your world and be seen in the way you should be seen. I want you to feel confident to step into new opportunities and try new things, so you don't live a life of regret or question if you shoulda, coulda, woulda.

We treat cash like it's king. You can do anything with cash. Well, you can't buy confidence, and confidence is the key to get you everything in life-- including money. Money can't buy you happiness, peace, love, success, relationships, but confidence will help you get all of those things. I want you to be as powerful as the queen in the game of chess, the one that can make the moves and can win the game. It's internal empowerment that will revolutionize your life, and the best part-- it's free! If you're ready to take control and live limitlessly- then buckle up- because we're about to fire it up!

~~~

It's probably easy to look at me and think I've always had confidence. I mean, I walk into places and people think I'm the owner- I've just got that vibe, I suppose! I walk in as a 6'1" woman with 4" heels and I tower over people. Literally, I walk in a room and eyes start coming my way. It's always been this way; the stares, I mean.

People have always finger-pointed, talked about my height, asked about my height, stared at me, taken pictures of me or with me. It's interesting to be me, no doubt! Today, my height is one of my greatest assets, but it was a journey, believe you me!

I remember as a child getting called the Jolly Green Giant, being asked *how's the weather up there?* I never had pants long enough and my mom always had to take the hem out of the pants I could find. It seemed hard to be tall. It was different being tall. It was uncomfortable being tall. I seemed to be one of the only tall females. I'm dating myself, but I lived before the Internet was made public. I didn't know tall women existed! I was even around before the WNBA (Women's National Basketball Association) came into existence! I don't know where the tall women were, but I certainly didn't come across many, and I felt seriously alone!

I learned at a young age just how uncomfortable growing pains can be. Yes, I mean the actual pains of growing. I grew almost half-a-foot in two years, and I can remember having sore legs and a back full of red lines. My aunt was a nurse and my mom had her take a look at my back one time. What were these unusual marks all over my lower back? Stretchmarks, that's exactly what they were. I grew so quickly that my skin couldn't keep up, and not even my mom knew what was going on (I'm the tallest in my family).

Kids can be cruel. How they ever got this way- I'm not totally sure, but they can be mean. I wish there were more anti-bullying initiatives and mindset classes when I was a kid, that would have been exceedingly helpful to get through life. But it seems we just figure out how to survive as we navigate through this playground called life. All I knew is I felt different, kids told me I was different, and I hated it.

"Why do you wear heels?"

"I don't want to stand next to you."

"Don't you think you're tall enough?"

"You're an amazon."

"You're too tall to ride this ride."

Yeah, kids can be really mean. It's hard enough trying

to navigate life while learning to accept your body, learn yourself, find friends, go to school, learn to date, manage your hormones, control your emotions, and then to be told you're different! Growing up was a rollercoaster!

My confidence was not high. There wasn't much I could do about my height, but I did try to make myself shorter, I absolutely tried. I remember thinking about every way I could shave the bone in my heels to make myself shorter. I had heard about women in Asia having surgery on their feet to fit into pointy-toed shoes, so there had to be a way for me to shave the bottom of my feet! But I was 12, how I was going to make that happen? So, I learned the hip lean.

The hip lean?

Yeah, you know that thing where you bump your hip out and you get shorter by an inch? Yes, that's what I did. My friend, Lisa, called me *Shelf* because she could rest her elbow on my hip. It took me from being a towering six-foot-one to six-foot. Wow, lots of good that did me! I ended up giving myself scoliosis. Now, as an adult I have a curved spine. Brilliant. You fooled the world for a few years that you were an inch shorter and now you have a permanently curved spine! Lesson learned there (and a reason we need to be mindful what we do to our bodies at a young age- let's add that to the grade school education)!

I really fought my height and I think I subconsciously tried to do things to distract people's attention. I don't know if me having bleach blonde hair, 19 piercings, and two tattoos by the time I was 17 years old had any correlation to how I felt about myself, but I'm pretty sure it did.

I was always into creating distractions. Look over here! Look at how amazing things look on the outside! While in the meantime, I hid my feelings and engaged in destructive behaviors that I kept hidden. I internalized everything people said to me. I didn't want to look weak, so I bottled up my feelings and shoved them under the rug. Not only did I internalize what people said, but I truly believed my height was a curse.

The truth is, I saw myself as nothing but flaws; my height, my weight, my personality, the size of my feet! I was a victim. The world was against me.

Had you told me the universe was always working for me and I had a choice of how I experienced this life I would have said you were crazy.

Let me tell you, that young girl didn't walk into establishments and people think she was the owner. Not even close! That girl didn't have the confidence to look at herself in the mirror and tell herself that she mattered, that she was loved, that she was valued. That girl had no value, so why would the world appreciate her when she didn't appreciate herself? She couldn't fathom the universe working for her. Unbeknownst to her, she gave away control over how she experienced life. So many people do.

It took me 35-years to figure out the way to win in life. I can honestly tell you that I'm grateful it only took me that long because some people never figure it out. Some people get to their deathbed and wonder what their life would be like if they had lived differently. I wouldn't have changed any of my journey either. I needed every step to get me to the moment I made a new choice in how I wanted to show up in the world.

Yesterday is gone. Every moment is a new moment to start over, and that's exactly what I did. May 13, 2018, I made the choice to change my world, to transform my life, to become the person I knew existed inside. That day changed my life forever. I was told the seven words that took me from victim to victor.

"You need to learn to love yourself."

Sounds so simple, but I had been fighting who I was for so many years. I kept seeking solutions for my problems, but I was looking externally to find the answers. How do I find happiness? How do I find success? How do I find peace? How do I find joy? How do I find meaningful relationships? How do I fix my problems and take control of my life? I tried all different external solutions—you know, the *how*. Nothing worked.

Why?

I went after temporary solutions instead of getting down to the root cause. The problem wasn't my height. The problem wasn't my drinking. The problem wasn't my eating disorder. The problem wasn't my divorce. The problem wasn't my job. The problem wasn't the men I dated. Every solution I found how to fix my problem was only temporary; until I finally looked in the mirror. I had a mindset problem.

On my journey to find self-love, I realized that everything I needed was already inside of me. I didn't understand the woman in the mirror. I didn't know how to love the woman in the mirror. I didn't know what the woman in the mirror was capable of. I didn't know the woman in the mirror was responsible for everything in her life. When I understood that life was a combination of mindset plus action, life changed. Everything I ever wanted became evident with that new piece of knowledge. The woman in the mirror that I avoided for my entire life was the answer to every problem I ever faced. I had to learn to trust her, to believe her, to have faith in her. Trust, belief, faith— that's the definition of confidence.

Finding the solutions to your problems might not look the way you think it's going to look. In this book we're going to uncover the way to get you to your most powerful state of being. You'll be able to dial in to your confidence and it will change your life. It's not the how to get to your solutions, we're focused on the way to find the answers, which are all already inside of you.

If there was some magic pill strategy, then that person would be a billionaire. I've spent thousands and thousands of dollars chasing resolutions. I tried so many external solutions of how to fix my problems; moving, shopping, Chinese Herbs, hypnosis, acupuncture, even thinking that if I got into a relationship then that would bring me happiness and all my problems would go away. You know what all those did? I had temporary happiness in my life. Pills don't give you skill. External solutions only give you temporary fixes. Period. The only way to make true change in your life and find your answer is to know yourself.

All the money I could have saved chasing solutions when I had what I needed the whole time!

Cash may be king, but it won't build your mind. It won't bring you long-term happiness. It won't give you confidence to do, to be, to get the life you want.

What I was missing every time I sunk money into a new *how to fix* solution? I wasn't getting honest with myself.

Why didn't I want to get honest?

It felt weird. I hated feelings. I had a lot of shame. My past was too littered with failures and let-downs. Who wants to do the work when you can just go shopping, or get in a relationship, or find some other distraction? Just fix the problem and move on, right? I didn't want to face myself, so I didn't. The result? My problems kept showing up again and again.

When I was 15 years old, my parents put me in modeling school. I remember graduating from John Casablanca's Modeling School and thinking I was going to make a career of modeling. Well, that didn't happen. Why? I didn't love myself. I didn't embrace myself. Who wants to take pictures of a woman who lacks confidence? Maybe a Prozac commercial would have wanted me.

It took me 20 year after graduating from modeling school for me to get comfortable in front of a camera. And now, as a hobby I work with photographers taking photos. I love it! It brings me so much joy to create art!

What's happening on the inside reflects on the outside. You can't fully hide it, even if you think you can. Your anger, your fears, your frustrations, your anxiety, your lack of confidence, your lack of self-love will all shine on the outside. Suffering is the external sign that there's internal work to do. It's amazing how many of us are wearing our emotions and problems out on our sleeves and not realizing it. Suffering is everywhere!

Suffering will be the roadblock keeping you from your solution. You are not in your most powerful state of being when you're in fear, frustrated, anxious, resentful, embarrassed, angry, tired, upset, or bored. You can't have clarity and flow when you have a clogged drain. You will have fluid motion in your life when you're connected to yourself. You are the motor in your vehicle. When your motor is running with trust, faith, and belief in yourself then you can take that car anywhere!

Confidence doesn't come naturally to everyone, but it's inside everyone. It's a journey. It's a process. It's something you practice. Once you've figured out how to tap into it, you've tapped into limitless potential. The world is your oyster. When you believe in yourself, when you trust who you are, when you believe everything is going to be OK then you have discovered life's wishing well.

You will continue to face things you've never faced. You will continue to step into new territory. Your life will continue to evolve, and as you do, it will require you to step into a new level of consciousness and confidence. Until you take your last breath you will be on this journey of evolving. You'll need to assess who you are, where you are, where you're going, and adapt as things change. This life isn't stagnant, so it's important you can bob and weave and keep that motor going toward your goals.

They say cash is king. You can do anything with cash, right? Well, I'll tell you, cash can't buy confidence. But confidence, well, that's the foundation you need to tackle everything. When you have confidence, you can do everything—including make money. So, which one is more powerful, the king or the queen?

The queen is the most powerful and coveted piece in a game of chess. She can move any number of squares in any direction. This is my goal for you. I want you to increase your confidence so you become the most powerful player in your world. I want you to find the way to your solutions. I want you to own the power moves.

Let's go, queens!

> *"All anything takes, really, is confidence."*
>
> — Rachel Ward

Chapter 2: What Exactly is Confidence?

If you start to pay attention to advertising, you find that advertisers believe that we, the consumer, want confidence.

British Airway's slogan is, "Flying with Confidence." Yes, I agree, I want confidence in the plane and pilot when I'm 35,000 feet in the air.

USA Pawn and Jewelry says, "Shop with Confidence," and I would also agree that I want confidence in jewelry from a pawn shop, so I don't get sold junk.

As James Monroe Homes says, "Build with Confidence," and I would agree that I need to be confident in my home builder. The last thing I need is for my home to fall apart.

The Swindon Borough Council says we need to "Eat with

Confidence," and that makes perfect sense because I want to know where my food comes from since I put it in my body.

Google any verb and put *with confidence* at the end. Sell. Perform. Insure. Exercise. Talk. Cook. Ride a bike. Answer the phone. Enhance your self-esteem. It doesn't matter what verb you use, you'll find a hit on how to do it with confidence. The world is telling us that we want to have confidence no matter what we are doing.

I often think confidence is this word we use from time-to-time when we want to do something big. It's something we tap into when we want to tackle something out of the ordinary; asking someone out, starting a business, asking someone to marry you, wearing that bathing suit you don't normally wear. I don't disagree that any of those take confidence, but I do believe we tend to overlook that _everything_ we do takes confidence.

Did you think about the last time you stood up? I didn't- I just did it. I've been standing up for almost 40 years, I don't put much thought into it (other than when I'm trying to get out of a small car, and I have heels on- that's not easy!). I also have strong legs. They've supported me through thousands and thousands of miles over the years. I'm an avid walker and runner and, although my knee pains me from time-to-time, I know when I stand-up, I walk. I know when I start to

22

run, I run. It was practice. The more I did it, the more confident I became. Now, it's not something I think about, I just have the confidence they'll do what they've always done. What if one day my legs aren't as strong?

As we age, our bodies change. This is why there tend to be railings, walkers, wheelchairs, and canes in the homes of seniors. As we age, our bodies deteriorate. Today, I don't get nervous to stand. I don't worry if I might fall backwards. As I age, that level of confidence might change as my body changes. I might have to be more careful as I stand and sit. Doesn't mean I can't have confidence in my ability to stand up and sit down, but I might not be able to do it without the assistance of someone or something.

I remember when I entered a hula-hoop contest when I was a kid. I was not the most athletic child and it was not something that came naturally for me. I do have a competitive mindset and I like to push myself. I think I was eight when we had this competition in grade school. My mom will tell you how I practiced my little heart out. Needless to say, when I started, I was not very good. I did not have the groove down and the hoop would fall within seconds of me starting to twirl. With some practice, I actually managed to keep it up! And with a little more practice, I gained the confidence in my skills. I ended up winning a blue ribbon for my whirling dervish moves (or maybe it was just a participation ribbon). I was ecstatic! All I needed was some practice to gain the confidence within myself.

Do you remember every detail about the last time you drove to the grocery store? Did you use a GPS? Probably not. You've been driving for so many years and you know where the grocery store is that you likely went on mental autopilot. You were confident in your driving and where you were going.

I remember when I was learning to drive. Going on Interstate-I66 was so scary. It's one thing to drive on a two-lane road, or around a parking lot, but merging on to a four-lane road in busy Northern Virginia can be really scary! I don't think I even used my side-view mirror. I cocked my head all the way around to look behind me. I didn't have the confidence to only use the tiny mirror hanging off the side of the car. I was much more trusting in my eyesight. God forbid there were blind spots and I hit someone (and this was way before cars got fancy and had internal cameras and noises that went off when you were merging close to someone). My trust was in my eyes. They hadn't failed me yet and I was a lot more confident in them than some itty-bitty side-view mirror. With time, using the mirror became effortless. I learned to find the blind spots. I learned how to correctly position the mirror. I understood the distance of the cars in the lane next to me so I could time switching lanes better. It took practice, but at some point, I stopped relying on just my eyes and I began to be confident in the mirror and my abilities.

What about your heartbeat? Ever even thought about it? Most of us when we're younger don't give it a second thought. We have healthy hearts. As we age, things can change. Or, as we modify our diets or our activity levels then the health of our heart can change. I personally don't think a whole lot about my heart. I have confidence it's going to do the job it needs to do to keep me alive. Repetition and consistency will give you confidence.

If you are someone that is overweight, eats a lot of fried food, has a sedentary lifestyle, is older, you may not have the same level of confidence in your heart's ability. Your doctor may tell you that you are high risk, or you may need a transplant, or a defibrillator, or a bypass, or to change your diet, or to start exercising. I guarantee you'll have a different level of confidence in the ability of your heart until you get cleared from the doctor.

Confidence is in everything. It's not just the big things, it's in every small thing you do. It's in people, places, things, ideologies.

Ever had a car that was on its last legs? Were you confident it was going to get you to work?

How about that co-worker that rarely pulls through on their deliverables? How confident are you that they're going to get their work in on time, and not impact *your* work?

What about going for a late lunch at 4pm? Are you confident that the restaurant is even open at that time or should you check the schedule to make sure they're still serving?

When you go into the restroom, you have confidence that when you go to the stall that there will be toilet paper. If there is not, that's a problem that you didn't expect.

When you go ice fishing, you should be confident about the ice not breaking below you.

When you buy something, anything, you should be confident that it's not broken.

Confidence is *everything*. This is why we find it in marketing so often. You want confidence that what you are spending money on is a proven and trustworthy product. If this is something you expect from your products, don't you think this is something you should also have within yourself? Don't you think people want this from you too?

Bigger topic than you realized, huh? I never really thought about the magnitude of confidence until it I went on my own quest to build it within myself. The more I explored the topic the more I realized that it was the core of everything.

As I started to brand myself as a Transformation & Confidence Coach, I noticed that not everyone believed they needed confidence. This goes back to people wanting to know how to solve their problems, and not realizing the way to do it is through confidence.

It wasn't confidence they needed, but rather better self-esteem, self-love, deeper relationships, how to build a business, or where to find happiness. As I tuned in what people's beliefs were about confidence, I acknowledged there was a disconnect. They just wanted to know *how*.

Another observation I made was that some people thought the way to get confidence was to surround yourself with confident people. Whereas I agree with that on many levels, it will only get you so far. Confidence is an inside job. Any exterior approach is a temporary one that won't get you that far.

I also came across many, many people that never thought about confidence as a mindset. It was something you had or you didn't. It was almost as if it was given to you at birth, not developed throughout your life. Practice may help some, but a lot of people didn't believe confidence was attainable by choice and had nothing to do with mindset.

Carol Dweck, a professor at Stanford University, did a study and found people fall in one of two categories. Either they have a growth or a fixed mindset. If you have a growth mindset then you are limitless in what you can do. You embrace opportunities. You don't place blame for the reason things didn't work out, but rather you take ownership. You believe that you can grow and stretch to the next level.

A fixed mindset is just the opposite. Whatever you are

born with is all you'll ever have, there is no growth. You don't see opportunities, you see roadblocks. You place blame when things don't work out.

These are two very different mindsets. If you have a fixed mindset, and you run into a roadblock, then you're likely to stop. You aren't telling yourself that if you practice more then you'll grow.

I saw a coach post recently on Facebook that mindset doesn't matter, but rather it's action that's important. I would argue that mindset comes before action. You need to believe in yourself and what you're doing to get into action. What keeps you going forward if you don't believe in yourself and what you're doing? What gets you through when the going gets tough? Mindset is foundational. It's your belief if you can or cannot. When you believe then you can achieve. Belief fuels actions. It will impact how you show up in the world, the risks you take, your self-esteem, how you see yourself.

If you try something and it doesn't work out, there can be one of two reactions. It can crush you or it can inspire you. This is fixed versus growth mindset, which Carol states we are all one or the other. If you feel crushed, you don't have a high self-esteem. If you're inspired to get up and do it again, this means you believe in yourself.

I go back to the conversations I've had with people that

said they didn't need confidence, but rather they just needed a better self-esteem. I'm not sure how these two can be isolated from each other?

Confidence is a state of certainty, a self-assurance within yourself.

It's the ability to feel secure in who you are.

It's not comparing yourself to others.

It's the feeling of being comfortable in your own skin.

It's a belief in knowing that everything is going to be OK.

It's being authentic to who you are.

It's acceptance and embracing yourself for everything you are and are not.

Confidence is trust.

Confidence is belief.

Confidence is feeling complete.

Imagine if you had all of these qualities. How do you think your self-esteem would be if you trusted and believed in yourself? The definition of being whole and complete is self-love. Wouldn't you have deeper relationships with others if you had a loving and secure relationship with yourself? Don't you need belief in yourself if you want to build a business? All roads, no matter what discussion I had, all led me back to confidence, but this idea seemed to be lost on so many people. They didn't need confidence, they just needed results. But how do you get the actions and results without the mindset? It's like asking for a house, but not wanting a foundation.

Confidence is a culmination of tools, practices, and ways of thinking. All roads lead back to needing confidence to achieve, to do, to be, to try, to buy anything. Confidence is the queen play, it's the most powerful positioning you can have.

~~~

I think about the children's movie, Cinderella. What a picturesque story that was! I'm sure every little girl probably dreams of being Cinderella and living that fairytale life. A prince swoops in and picks you up off your feet and gives you a life you could only dream about. Truth is, you have more chance in winning the lottery (but it happened to Meghan Markle- so never say never).

Although the movie was cute and gave all little girls hope of a prince charming, there was something much deeper happening in the movie. Cinderella didn't have a glamorous life. She was merely the maid. She wasn't appreciated by her family and her stepsisters were mean to her. They made her do the cleaning and she wasn't allowed to be a part of the family activities. They created a hierarchical system within the family and they decided she was going to be at the bottom. They were going to be their mother's favorite.

Despite being suppressed by her sisters, Cinderella kept a relatively positive attitude. She cleaned, did her chores with a smile, and even made some little mouse friends along the way that loved and supported her. It would have been easy for Cinderella to bite back at her sisters, sabotage them when they were sleeping, poison their food, but she didn't.

It's not always easy to take the high road, but there's definitely less traffic. It's easier to get negative, to retaliate, get down on yourself, curl up in a ball. It's much harder to stand up when you feel defeated. It's much harder to walk away from friends that gossip about you and not do the same back to them. It's much harder to find the strength within yourself when the going gets tough. If you can, you've found the road less traveled, the ones that are on the path to peace, clarity, love, and confidence.

This is precisely why Cinderella didn't bite back at her sisters. She had confidence and self-love. She was at peace. She had clarity of her own value and knew she wasn't defined by how her sister's saw her.

When someone has confidence and self-love then they aren't lacking anything. It's like a sponge that is full of water; it can't soak up anything more than what it already has. The sponge is full of positivity, happiness, clarity, confidence, gratitude, peace. It didn't matter what her sister's said, she was that full sponge, she didn't have space in life to take on any of their thoughts or opinions. In fact, her positivity polarized their negativity.

She wasn't going to be defined by her sisters. She wasn't going to be hateful just because her sisters were. She wasn't going to perceive herself as less just because her sister's did. Cinderella stayed in her lane and nothing changed her perception, her value, her self-worth because she already knew who she was. She knew she was princess potential!

In fact, not only was she not impacted by her evil sisters, she continued to have hope, lived in gratitude, and stayed positive! This is what a full sponge looks like.

Put yourself in Cinderella's shoes (not the glass slippers, but rather the ratty ones she wore to clean). Do you think you would have reacted the same way she did? This situation is a breeding ground for anger, resentment, frustration, none of which are the higher road. You might feel betrayed and wonder why your stupid, ugly stepsisters get all the special treatment. You might get jealous that they get to attend fancy events while you hang out with the mice and clean the house. What kind of life is that? I'm sure that's how many of us might feel. It's much harder to be grateful, to pick your head up and keep going, to value yourself when others are devaluing you.

Confidence is a feeling of the full sponge. When you aren't full, when you aren't whole, you'll find this is where betrayal, jealousy, resentment, anger, anxiety reside. Cinderella wasn't comparing herself to her sisters. Rather, she was focused on herself. When the opportunity presented itself for her to go to the ball, she didn't question if she was good enough, she believed she was. Cinderella remained true to who she defined herself as. And, her confidence shined though. The prince saw it and he knew she was the one.

Authenticity is confidence. How good does it feel to be in the comfort of your own home? Imagine if you could share that person with the world and accept who you are and not care what others think?

I always worked in a male-dominated industry, information technology, and I never felt as though I could be my true self. I had this idea, first and foremost, that there's a corporate persona, and if I wanted to survive, then I needed to fit the cookie cutter mold like everyone else. Secondly, because I was working with all men, I felt that I had to adapt to the male way of doing things. I also didn't want to be viewed for my femineity because I thought it would take away from how smart the men would view me. I would wear my hair up, so it didn't flow down to my mid-back. I stopped wearing earrings, so I didn't have anything distracting near my face. I didn't want to wear tight clothing because I didn't want the men to see my figure. I wanted my mind to be seen, and in order to do this, I thought I needed to be like one of the guys.

That was the furthest thing from being authentic to who I really was. I felt like Fiona from Shrek, "By day one way, by night another." It was two very different lives and quite honestly it was exhausting. Now, I realize there is always going to be a difference between how you act in an office and in your home. I don't want to be professional at home and I certainly don't want to fart in front of my coworkers or clients. So yes, there is likely always going to be standards within the home that vary from the standards in a professional environment. When I talk about authenticity, I'm talking about someone who isn't afraid to be who they are at the core.

I was absolutely not being authentic to myself. I don't care about baseball. Don't care about golf. Don't like to wear my hair up. Don't like baggy clothing. Don't like wishing I would get invited to happy hours with the guys, but not feeling I could speak up to say I wanted an invite. I wondered far too often why my peers went to lunch together, but never would include me. This was not being authentic to myself and not someone that exhibited a high degree of confidence. I was a sponge that wasn't full. I was more jealous of my coworkers than an equal, in my mind, anyhow. I didn't value myself enough to speak up or stand up for myself.

When you don't know who you are, it's easy to adapt to your surrounding to make yourself fit in or pick someone you want to be like. This is the opposite of authenticity and is contrary to confidence. How can you be confident when you aren't being you?

A past girlfriend of mine told me once that she changes herself to match the likes and dislikes of the guy she's dating. She told me this was her strategy to get guys to like her. She also thought it made her a *good girlfriend* because he wouldn't have to compromise anything.

After the vomit in the back of my throat went down, I was able to think further about the words she had just told me. It's not my job to go around telling people my opinions or fix everyone (being a coach there's a fine line I walk), but in my mind a lot of things were happening.

If you're willing to change yourself for someone, why would they want to pick you? If you are going to mirror someone, is that what they want? I don't know that a guy wants to date a version of himself. Granted, I acknowledge there will be the fundamental differences between a male and a female, but is a guy looking for someone that does and says yes to everything he wants? Is a guy looking for a bobble-head of a girlfriend, or one of those people from work that that yes to everything? Don't guys like women with hobbies and interests? Maybe not a narcissist, but is that what we're going after here?

If the man changes his likes and dislikes, do you also continue to change and adapt? I can't imagine this to be attractive. If someone only wants eye-candy (someone that's good looking) and doesn't care about substance, then yes, I can see this working (and that's what this woman was, eye candy).

My biggest issue with this woman's approach was that it exhibited zero self-confidence in herself for what she brought to the table. She completely dismissed who she was as a person. That's not sexy. She was basically saying she didn't matter and wasn't valuable. He was worth far more and therefore she should change herself for him. I always struggled with watching this, and, for the record, her relationships never lasted.

You are the only you. You are the only one that can be you. Stepping into your authentic self is such a special thing that no one else can be or do for you!

I think of how many stories I've heard of people showing up on dates from an online dating service and they don't look like their picture they took ten years before. It's called *catfishing*. I've never heard of one of those dates ending well. The person that feels they were catfished feels lied to, and they don't feel the person was being true and authentic.

When someone isn't true and authentic to themselves, what else are they hiding? I personally didn't feel good when a guy lied about his age by nine years. Come to find out, he had a lot more under the surface that he was hiding.

~~~

Confidence is like having a security blanket. Trust. Belief. Feeling complete. Being authentic. Secure. Being at home with yourself. Certainty. It's knowing that everything is going to be OK. When you have confidence, you're that sponge that doesn't need anything else. You're that sponge full of positivity, you're complete, negativity can't penetrate you.

Confidence doesn't just exist with the big things; it exists with *everything*! From breathing and walking to marriage proposals and starting a company. Everything in life can be boiled down to confidence. That's why William Hazlitt said, "As is our confidence, so is our capacity." You are only capable of doing what you are confident doing.

As we go through this book, I want you to start to open your mind to the idea that confidence is everything and everything needs confidence to thrive. You'll learn how to boost your confidence and how to change the way you see things. Become that sponge.

You are unstoppable. You are limitless! It's already inside of you.

Now, go turn on the song by Demi Lovato, *Confident*, and let that authentic side of you bubble to the surface!

"As is our confidence, so is our capacity."

-William Hazlitt

Chapter 3: What does Confidence Feel Like?

That Demi Lovato's song, *Confident*, gets me every time! I don't know about you, but I start walking the model's catwalk around my apartment when that song comes on! It's instantaneous confidence whenever it's playing!

Imagine you have confidence. Sit with that feeling for a bit. You have the trust, belief, love, security within yourself. What does it feel like? Warm? Bold? Strong? Comfortable? Exciting? Secure? Safe?

How different does your daily routine feel with confidence? Sit with that feeling.

Let's get really clear on what you imagine confidence looking and feel like in your own life. This way, when it shows up you'll know what it is. Manifest how you imagine your life changing.

If you're lost, think of someone you know that has confidence. What do you think they feel? How do they show up and act in situations? I think of women like Brene' Brown, Julia Haart, and Jennifer Vaughan.

Brene' is comfortable with who she is as a person. She jokes. She's not afraid to be vulnerable. She has no reservation or intimidation bantering with Oprah. She stands behind her research and the messages she gives to the world. She doesn't try to change her accent, look like one of Hollywood's blonde chicks, or hide her cursing when she gives a presentation. Brene' is unapologetically herself.

Julia Haart made a bold lifestyle change after she turned 40 years of age. This tenacious woman is an absolute firecracker. She knows what she wants and she's not afraid to go after it. After leaving her Orthodox Jewish way of life and husband, she built a shoe company and then took over as CEO of Elite World Group in New York. In less than 10 years, Julia went from a rather oppressive lifestyle to ultimate freedom. She wears miniskirts, runs a successful company, and her life is on a reality TV show! Spunky! She knows what she wants, she loves who she is, and she dreams limitlessly. Julia is authentically Julia. Period.

I personally adore Jennifer Vaughan. I found Jennifer after discovering a YouTube video of her one Saturday night. Jennifer has HIV and has gone public with her story. She is hands-down one of the most inspiring and self-confident people I have ever met. To come out to the world with something so stigmatized and vulnerable is far too terrifying for most people to think about. Jennifer holds nothing back. I watch her videos because I love seeing her own her story and who she is. She even recently started dating and is sharing that journey. She openly talks about how people shun her, but she doesn't let it bother her. Jennifer is inspiration and strength. I love everything about her! She doesn't try to be anyone else other than who she is.

All three of these women exude confidence. All three have very different personalities, but at the core they have the same traits. They're self-aware, authentic, secure, believe in themselves, and they're in flow with their lives. Nothing can stop them!

What does confidence look like for you? We're not talking about being cocky. Get the used-car salesman idea out of your head and think about these amazing women.

Maybe you'd say NO more to things you don't want and YES to more things you do. How would that feel?

Maybe you'd wear that outfit that shows a little bit of skin. How would that feel?

Maybe you'd ask for a promotion. How would that feel?

Maybe you'd go on more dates. How would that feel?

Maybe you'd tell the waitress your food was cold instead of just eating it because you don't want to hurt anyone's feelings. How would that feel?

Maybe you would start that business you've talked about for years? How would that feel?

Maybe you'd find a new group of friends because you know your current group is soul sucking and not supportive. How would that feel?

Maybe you'd explore the world more. How would that feel?

I hope you at least feel empowered. Confidence is empowering.

Close your eyes and really think about the changes that you would make within your life if you had confidence. What feeling would come with those changes? Zig Ziglar said so eloquently, "if we aim at nothing, we hit our target every time." If we don't know where we are going, then we are aimlessly moving through life.

I lacked a lot of confidence when it came to my height. I knew I wanted to feel comfortable with who I was. I wanted to look in the mirror and have that warm feeling of love and admiration. You know, that feeling of sitting by the fire or eating some warm mac & cheese on a cold winter's night? I wanted to feel that way about myself.

I wanted to walk in a room and not feel like I was ogre towering over people. I wanted to embrace the comments they said to me and receive them with a grateful heart. I wanted to wear the shoes that made me feel sexy and not just the ones that made me less tall. That's how I wanted to feel. That's who I wanted to be. That's who I became.

Doesn't mean I don't have my days, but I know where I'm aiming. I know what I want to feel like. I know where I want to be. You need to get clear on the person you want to become and not just be the person you happened to become. Again, are you happening to life, or is life happening to you? It's time you take control of how your life looks, feels, and how you show up.

When you are confident then you have an assurance within yourself that everything is going to work out. You trust that everything is going to be OK no matter what. It feels like standing on a rock, you trust you are on solid ground.

How would it feel if you knew who you were? You knew what you liked, disliked, your values, your beliefs. Not only were you self-aware, but you also honored yourself and stayed true to what resonated with you. How amazing would it feel to show people the real you and not worry what anyone else thought? What if you were authentically you? This is opposite of the woman I mentioned in the last chapter who changed herself for any and every man. There's something magical that happens when you know yourself. Sun Tzu said, "know yourself and you will win all battles."

It's this level of awareness and connection within yourself that you're aiming for. It's this level of understanding and respect you want internally. It's knowing your strengths and your weaknesses. It's knowing your beliefs and your morals. This knowledge will help you navigate through your life. You give yourself permission to try. You give yourself permission to ask. You give yourself permission to delegate. You give yourself permission to do things that may not turn out the way you expected them to turn out. You can win any battle when you know who you are, respect, and honor yourself.

Confidence is the security in knowing that the world is working for you and not against you. Even when life doesn't pan out the way you thought it would, you know it all happened for a reason. It's a peaceful feeling when you know the world is in your court and each brick is strategically placed to help you advance and grow.

When I think about the general feelings of confidence, it's everything I believe people aspire to have in their own lives. We want the fruits of the spirit: love, joy, peace, patience, kindness, goodness, faithfulness, gentleness, and self-control. We want to be secure, to be comfortable, to be happy, to be respected, to be seen, to be acknowledged, to be ourselves. You experience these feelings when you are in a beautiful state being. This is the opposite of suffering. Suffering is something that happens to you, a beautiful state is something you choose.

Whenever I'm about to open the door to my apartment, I get this wave of bliss knowing that I'm about to see my cat, Booger. She's always so excited to see me, especially after a long trip. When she hasn't seen me for a few days, she loves to converse with me. She likes to tell me about all the PBS shows she was watching, she's a big fan of Bob Ross and his happy trees! She is the softest cat and her fur alone makes me happy! She's not big on me picking her up, but she tolerates it for 20-30 seconds. I love when she lets me snuggle with her. In the morning, she wakes me up with kisses on my face. It's weird, but I've grown to love her morning kisses. This is love. This is happiness. And in many ways, this is what confidence feels like-- bliss!

How about when you practice for something and you nail it! What a good feeling, right? It's that feeling of accomplishment! I remember getting my first truck. I grew up in an area where trucks were not prevalent, so I was entirely unfamiliar with them. I started with a Toyota Tacoma, which is a relatively smaller truck. You may have thought it would have been easy for me to manage, but it wasn't. I looked like Austin Powers trying to maneuver that thing.

The only way to figure it out was to practice. Although I was a bit foolish looking for a couple of months, I eventually leaned how to park without taking two minutes to inch my way into a spot. It was a feeling of accomplishment-- like getting that sticker from your grade school teacher.

Every time I traded in a truck, I seemed to upgrade the size (I want a monster truck one day- I'm speaking that into existence). I eventually owned a diesel Ford F-250 Super Duty with 35-inch wheels and a lift. It was beautiful and it was large! Every time I backed that vehicle into a spot and parked, I had this wave of accomplishment. Literally, every time! Best of all, was when I parked perfectly on the first try (which was most of the time- I'm just sayin'). I would say something like, *you GO girl*, because it felt that good. It was like high fiving myself and patting myself on the back. My practice gave me confidence, and my confidence felt like that of a little schoolgirl getting her first kiss.

You know that t-shirt you wear that has been washed a million times and it's so soft and comfortable? You know, that one you wear to sleep or when you're lounging around the house. Confidence is like that kind of comfort!

I'm sure some happy memories have flooded your brain and you've found yourself going down your own rabbit holes of times when you were happy and felt good. Winning a prize. Childhood friends. Holidays. Laughing until you peed your pants. Losing track of time because you're engaged in such a good conversation. Getting asked out for the first time. Your first kiss. Your first child. Your pet. Chasing fireflies. Going on vacation. I hope you have experienced happiness in your life at some point and I hope you're experiencing those feeling now.

Confidence just feels good. It's like nothing else matters. It's just you in that moment!

Now, what if I told you to get naked and get in front of the mirror. Not the little, tiny mirror by the door where you check your teeth before you leave the house. I'm talking about the full-length mirror where you see everything. How do you feel? My hope is that you are in the 15% that are positive about how they feel about their bodies. Most of us fall in the 62% that are only accepting of what we see in the mirror. Then, there are 23% that are negative about what they see (Dold, K. (2017). This is How Women Today REALLY Feel About Getting Naked, *Women's Health Magazine*).

The truth is, getting naked can be really awkward for many people. When we put clothes on then we are able to cover up the creases and the folds and the ignore the fact that we don't have abs and might have some flab. Out of sight, out of mind. This exercise of getting confident may feel a bit like standing naked in that mirror. Growth is usually uncomfortable, but it's the only way. It's getting honest with yourself about where you are, it's acknowledging where you want to be, and it's coming up with a plan on how to get there.

You may very well not want to see yourself standing there naked. It may make you feel uncomfortable to the point that you want to put clothes on and go back to what you know. It's normal. Know where you want to go and you'll get there. It takes you getting honest with yourself, it's the only way.

If you are looking to make a change, know that these feelings will arise. It's the storm before the rainbow. Don't let your brain trick you to go backwards. Take control. Focus on your goals. Stand up for where you want to be, who you want to be, and how you want to feel. There is no one that can do this work for you and change doesn't happen by chance.

You are in full control of your destiny, your happiness, how you want to feel, how you want to show up in this world. Only you stand up for what you want.

Confidence is the most amazing and beautiful state of being that you can be in, if you do the work.

Keep your mindset on how you want to feel and don't let that brain trick you back to where you started.

"The most beautiful thing you can wear is confidence."

-Blake Lively

Chapter 4: Your Journey

Before we dive into the world of confidence, let's get real clear on what it is not. I often hear someone describe a person they've labeled as confident, yet they're characterizing someone that's arrogant and pompous. Being confident and being cocky can easily be mixed up, but there's a world of difference between the two. You need to know where you're going before you start heading in any particular direction.

Two guys are having a drink at the bar and a handsome guy walks in by himself. He comes strolling in through the doors, shoulders back, and a long stride. He walks directly over to the opposite end of bar where he believes no one is waiting for a drink. He looks the bartender in the eyes, smiles, asks how he's doing, and orders a drink.

A smaller woman next to him says, "Hey, I was waiting."

The guy immediately says he's sorry and tells the bartender to get her order first. "Sorry, I didn't realize you were waiting. My apologies."

After the woman gets her drink, he orders his beer and takes a seat in a corner while he plays on his phone.

Does this sound confident or cocky?

The two guys at the end of the bar watch the transaction and one says, "What a cocky jerk! Didn't even see that girl waiting for her drink! He probably drives a big truck and is trying to compensate for something. What a schmuck."

What do you think?

It's true, the guy may not have seen the woman waiting, but that could have been an honest mistake. He did immediately correct the situation and even apologized. He also appeared to go to an area of the bar that didn't seem to have anyone waiting. A long stride, shoulders back, and making eye contact doesn't entirely mean he's cocky.

Let's look at some of the key differences between being confident and cocky (or arrogant).

Confident	Cocky
Self-assurance	Exaggerated sense of importance
Will talk to strangers	Stays around familiar faces
Admits ignorance	Shows off being right
Not afraid to act silly	Afraid to not be taken seriously
Talk to powerful people to sell ideas	Talk to powerful people to be seen
Willing to learn	Knows everything
Willing to listen	Doesn't want to be told
Highlight and praise others	Talk about and praise themselves
Don't brag	Boast about achievements
Attract people to them	Polarize people
Aware of giving others space to talk	Talk over people
Internal validity	**External validity**

Someone that is cocky has something to prove. They're

so afraid of being wrong or seen as unsuccessful that they will go to great lengths to be right and appear successful. They want to be seen around the elite and want to look important. Someone that's cocky needs external validation.

What about the guy ordering a drink? Was he cocky or not? He was willing to listen, willing to admit he was wrong, and wasn't afraid to be seen alone. From this small example, I'd say he was confident. He may have just made an honest mistake and legitimately may have thought this woman was hanging out at the bar not waiting to order.

By the end of this book, you're going to see how confidence is an inside job. It's not about having others validate you, it's about you being OK regardless of what is happening around you. It's self-assurance and not needing to rely on anyone. You own your success, your security, your happiness, your progress, and you hold the keys to the kingdom.

We tend to have respect for people with confidence. A confident leader is someone we would want to follow. They're sure of their direction, they are willing to listen, willing to learn, they give praise where praise is due. Confident people are generally positive and pleasant to be around.

In 2013, the National Court Reporters Association came out with an article that stated "Those who possess high self-confidence tend to be more positive, and for this reason, they attract more positivity into their lives. Because of this, self-confident people tend to be overall happy and fulfilled individuals." Who doesn't want to be around someone that is positive and happy? Confidence is a magnet; people gravitate towards this energy. It also sexy. Someone that is secure with who they are and aren't always tearing themselves or others down is an attractive quality to have.

Confidence is when you believe in yourself and your abilities, arrogance is when you think you are better than others and act accordingly.

-Stewart Stafford

~~~

When you think of someone that is confident, who comes to mind? When you look at the qualities listed here, is there someone you think of that you admire? What traits about that person do you find admirable?

What do you imagine your life looking like with more confidence?

Would you try new things? What would you try?

Would you explore new territories? Where would you go?

Would you walk into a room differently? How would it change?

How would you act at a party? Would you talk to more people? Would you dance?

Start to get a clear picture of what your life would look like if you had this thing called confidence.

What does it look like?

What does it feel like?

What changes in your life?

How do you show up differently?

What have you always wanted to do that you would now feel comfortable doing?

Would your relationships change? If so, how?

Lots of questions, but they're important.

Decide on what you want rather than what you don't want. When you strive for what you want then you're automatically going to weed out what you don't. Focus on that positive energy and that's what you'll attract.

You're making the intentional decision to change your life and maybe even how you see yourself. You get to decide how you show up and what you'll find is that the mind plays a huge role in how you see everything. The mind doesn't know how to differentiate between an idea and the truth. Start to train your brain to see what you want to see so you can become who you want to become.

You may not feel confident about talking to strangers but start telling yourself you are.

You might be nervous to dance in front of strangers but tell yourself it's fun and you love to let loose!

Training the brain is a skill. You can literally become anything you want if you put your mind to the task.

~~~

Every time you level up in your life, reach a new stage, become a bit more wise or mature, the way you see the world is going to change. With new knowledge you may make new decisions. With new beliefs you will have different experiences. Each new level you reach requires a new you.

Let's say your business starts to grow. You were a six-figure company and now you're operating at a seven figures. The demand is different. You'll need more employees or more automation. You may be required to provide a different level of customer service. In order to attract top talent, you may need to offer different benefits to your employees. There may be different employment laws you need to comply with. To meet a higher demand, you will go through growth and changes. Same is true in your own life.

Imagine if everything in life was easy. Every process

came naturally. Happiness was easy. Money flowed. People would flock to buy your product or service without even having to advertise. You always nailed it on the first try. Don't you think everyone would have happiness and a million dollars in the bank? It sounds too good to be true because it is. Life isn't hard and it's not rocket science, but it's work. Many people aren't willing to do the work or they don't know they even have the option to change.

As you make the decision to level up your life, as you reach new heights and potential for yourself, it will come with unfamiliarity and even discomfort. Life is full of challenges, change, ups and downs. When you step into the unknown, it can feel like you're free falling. You've gone from secure footing to figuring out a new zone of genius. It's normal to feel out of place when you experience the new. It will likely come with discomfort. We'll talk later on about rewiring the brain and controlling your mind, but realize you have full control over how you interpret your experiences. Knowing and embracing the feelings associated with stretching yourself will help you embrace the process rather than turn around and run back to where you came from.

Back in 2009, I took an amazing trip with my ex-husband to Thailand. There are some of the most picturesque islands and beaches there. In 2000, the movie, *The Beach*, was filmed on the island of Ko Phi Phi Le with Leonardo DiCaprio, who plays the main character,

Richard. Richard sets out to find paradise, a place where he can find solitude, and he comes upon a beautiful beach. White sand, turquoise water, surrounded by mounds of earth, covered in moss and greenery jutting high out of the ocean creating a privacy-like wall around the magnificent beach. Heaven. It's what I'd imagine Heaven would look like.

My ex and I decided we were going to cliff jump in this heavenly spot. I'd never done this before, but I'm big on experiences and I love a good adrenaline rush. We took a boat to another island where the mounds of earth jut far out of the ocean into the sky. A group of us got to this piece of paradise and we made our way to the buffet lunch. Our excursion was all you could eat, jump, and drink. Not sure that's the wisest combination, but that's what our $50 package came with.

I'd love to say I was the first to dive off the cliff into the turquoise water, but I was most certainly not the first. In theory, I was ready to do something I had never done before, but when I saw the height of the diving board I lost my confidence. I had jumped off a diving board in the past. I may have even jumped from a board that was five to ten feet above the water, but I had never jumped into an ocean from 30-50 feet in the air. Conceptually, I could make the jump. When I saw how far down it actually was-- I froze.

I'm not promoting liquid courage to get over your fears

in life (drinking your way to confidence), but the package did include unlimited alcohol. After eating, watching, and drinking for a bit, I convinced myself I was ready. Other people had gone multiple rounds before I ever got started, and they survived! I was also starting to feel a bit more relaxed and courageous because of the mai tais I was drinking.

There I went. I told my ex I was ready. He grabbed my camera and watched me take off up the rocky mound. It felt like I was making my way to the end of a plank on a pirates ship, about to splash into the ocean. There was no running and jumping, I inched my way to the end of that plank that overlooked the sea from what felt like way up in the sky.

Can I do this?

Am I going to survive?

Will I hurt myself?

What if I hit something?

There were tons of questions that went around in my head, my confidence was about at a 2 on a scale of 1-10 (one being low and ten being high). And then I jumped. I remember the air as it wrapped around my body as I made my way towards the water. It felt like it took forever, even though it was probably only two or three seconds. Once I had lifted off, I left the fears, the feeling, my trepidation on the plank and I enjoyed the air rushing through my hair and the breeze against my soft skin.

And then...

Splash! I reached the water.

I remember intense feeling of smashing into the cold water. I did not have the grace of a diver or a swimmer. There were parts of me that hit the water without any grace at all, like my bum, and I felt it. I went far under the water and quickly back to the surface.

I did it! I jumped in the water and got back out, just like I was supposed to!

"How was it?!" my ex asked.

"Ah-maZING! I'm going to do it again!"

I made my way back to the plank, walked boldly to the end, and jumped off. No hesitation. No reservation. I was confident in what I was doing (granted I was fueled by mai tais as well, but I was the first time too). This time, I tucked my rear end, so it didn't feel like I landed on a firehose when I hit the water. Perfection! Or at least better than the first time!

When you're growing, you are stretching yourself, which can feel uncomfortable. There could be fear, pain, uncertainty. But we know that it's only after the storm that there comes a rainbow. When you are growing, you are going through a storm of learning something new. It can be exciting and scary at the same time. Your brain may even try to convince you to turn around and run back to where you came from. It's you making the conscious decision to move through the discomfort that will get you to the rainbow on the other side.

If you are starting a business, moving in with someone, entering into a new relationship, or putting a little extra hot sauce on your wings- there will be a new level of growth you'll experience.

If knowing is half the battle then you can better hold on to your confidence as you are entering into new waters, unchartered territories, experiencing the new. You will need to tell your mind that this is supposed to happen so that it doesn't revert backwards to what it knows.

Our brains are designed to keep us safe, and when it enters into new territory it says:

> *Warning, you've never done this, you don't*
> *know how it's going to end! Go back. Turn*
> *around. It's safe back there!*

That's when you politely step in the driver's seat and tell yourself it's going to be OK (yes, have a conversation with yourself). The universe is always working for you and it will adapt around you as you make new decisions.

As you start to grow, remember how you imagined your

life would look. Let that guide you. Remember how you felt as you became the person you envisioned. Be intentional about how you want to feel, who you want to be, and keep reminding yourself of that person as you enter each new stage of your development. Aim for that confident person.

As you grow, it will feel uncomfortable. Discomfort doesn't mean to turn around. Know that when you feel discomfort that you are growing. It's not a reason to shut down, but rather to keep going. You are becoming who you envisioned. Embrace the journey.

"Be not afraid of discomfort. If you can't put yourself in a situation where you are uncomfortable, then you will never grow. You will never change. You'll never learn."

-Jason Reynolds

Chapter 5: Knowledge is Power

It's important to understand at a high-level how the six inches in between your ears operates so you have a better understanding at a functional level how to navigate. Knowledge is power, so stick with me for a brief overview so you can grasp what is the brain, mind, and mindset, and how they play together. This is the only semi-technical chapter, but it's foundational. The more you know about how you're designed, then you can start to navigate your headspace and take control. The goal is to be in the driver's seat of your life. Many of us, are in the passenger seat and we don't even know it.

This was me. I was a passenger.

I was not aware that I had any input on if I was angry, mad, frustrated, resentful, enraged, anxious, and every other state of suffering. Situations would happen throughout my day and I would react without ever asking if that's how I wanted to feel. If those emotions and thoughts served me. I found myself in suffering constantly. This is being in the passenger seat.

If someone cut me off on the road, I got pissed off.

If my coworker said something stupid, I rolled my eyes.

If my friend canceled plans, I'd be irritated.

I realized that it didn't serve me to be in a negative state of mind and in suffering. I actually had a say in how I responded. If you asked me if I would rather be upset or at peace, I could tell you my answer. It became clear that my thoughts and actions didn't reflect how I would want to think and act if given the option. I had the option, I just didn't know it.

Life doesn't get to tell you how to respond, it's a right you own. The brain, the mind, and mindset are the foundation of creating the life you want. The life you want is in those six inches between your ears. It's like magic, if you know how to do the trick.

STICK WITH ME....it's not painful....I promise!

Brain

The brain is the squishy, arguably ugly looking organ that's found in your head. It's that wrinkly blob of mass that we protect with a helmet when we ride a bike. If this gets damaged in any way, it can impact how you talk, think, walk, and navigate life. It's the hub of your thoughts, which have paved the paths to your beliefs. Beliefs then drive behavior and habits.

Beliefs are influenced by how you grew up, the people you surround yourself with, what you listen to, your religion, the country you live in, your experiences, or your daily routine. There are so many factors that impact what you think, which then creates your beliefs, which then impacts behavior and habits. Since we all have different experiences in life, this lends itself to all different sets of beliefs and how to operate or react.

Imagine if you had an encounter with a big dog and it bit you. You may believe that big dogs are vicious. You may believe that cats are better than dogs because they can't bite as hard. You may believe that all dogs are scary. You may believe every dog wants to attack you. Your experience with the one dog could have led to any number of beliefs that you carry with you throughout your life.

You may not have been bitten by a dog, but maybe your parents always talked about how much they hated them when you were growing up. They told you dogs are scary, evil, and will bite you. When you see a dog, it's a natural reaction for you to be fearful of what they might do based off what your parents led you to believe.

Your friend may have had a bad experience and is

always talking about her fear when she sees a big dog. After hearing this on repeat enough, you too start to dislike dogs. You may think that, based off her experience, you too will have the same happen if you encounter a large dog. Your belief is that big dogs are frightening.

Your thoughts become your beliefs. That thought pattern is the path in your brain. If you change the way you think, then you can change your belief. When you change your belief then your experiences in life change. You can change the structure of your brain if you understand how to control your thoughts. This means, you need to consciously be aware of the messages you are ingesting and the thoughts you allow to filter through you.

I think of these pathways like the literal walking paths I take when I go in the woods. Ever walked through the woods where there are paths that people previously created? We tend to stay on the path that already exists. If we go off the beaten path, then there may be snakes hiding, debris in the way, or we may get lost, so we don't usually deviate.

It was once believed the pathways in your brain, called neuroplasticity, could not be changed once they were created (like no deviating from the paths in the woods). We now know, however, the brain absolutely can be rewired, remapped, reprogrammed. It's a muscle. Just like abs, with work and repetition, we can train this muscle to look any way we want! Rewiring the brain isn't something that happens overnight (same as getting six-pack abs), but recreating new pathways can be formed with the right training and diligence.

Additionally, the brain is connected to the spinal cord, which is like a telephone system talking to body and relaying information from the brain to the body.   The brain is the command center and the spinal cord disseminates the commands. Together, the brain and the spinal cord make up our Central Nervous System (CNS).

The CNS is responsible three things: sensing, processing, and output. Think of this a bit like Google. You put information or a request into Google's search engine, Google searches it's database, and spits out a result. Depending on what search criteria you use you may get a different output.

Back to the example of the dog. You see a dog, your brain searches for information. It thinks it's in danger because you believe all dogs are harmful because of your past experience. You turn and run because fear has taken over. If you didn't believe the dog was harmful then you wouldn't flinch.

Your brain is going to send a signal through your spinal cord and your motor skills will reflect what your brain is thinking.

Imagine if we were searching a database that had all

garbage in it. Ever heard of *garbage in, garbage out*? It's the same with our brains, which is why it's so important we feed it properly.

There are two ways of feeding the brain we'll touch on; foods you eat, and messages you send to your brain.

Foods that are high in saturated fats and sugar lead to poorer performance in the brain, which is why it's crucial you are feeding your body the proper food to then nourish your brain. Consuming excessive amounts of sugar impairs cognitive skills and self-control, and ultimately can damage your brain and result in other health issues, such as diabetes. We want the command center to be at its peak performance, so when it's communicating to the rest of the body through the spinal cord it's conveying a strong message.

Healthline suggests 11 foods to enhance your brain's activity and memory.

1. Fatty fish (like salmon)
2. Coffee (in moderation)
3. Blueberries
4. Turmeric
5. Broccoli
6. Pumpkin Seeds
7. Dark Chocolate
8. Nuts
9. Oranges
10. Egg
11. Green Tea

By adding these foods into your diet, you can help boost your memory, mood, alertness, and brain development.

Now, think of the messages and data you are sending to your brain everyday:

- Music
- Sounds
- Television
- What you read
- Conversations
    - Office
    - Home
    - Religious
    - Political
    - Friends
    - Affiliations/groups

From sun-up to sun-down you are constantly feeding your brain with messages. Just like the impact foods can have on your overall brain performance, same is true with what messages and data you are feeding your brain.

Have you ever heard someone speak and it sounds like they've been brainwashed?

We typically associate brainwashing with more extreme, radical forcing of information on to a person to get them to conform to a social, religious, or political beliefs. I think of the recruits for some of the Muslim extremist practices who blow up themselves to become martyrs, or those who followed Hitler, or people in Africa who believe having sex with a virgin will get rid of AIDS. These are extreme, but those who follow them believe them to be true. They have been influenced by radicals and their brain has programmed their beliefs, which then impacts how they react.

It seems extreme, but these people are no different than you and me. The difference is their beliefs, which have been influenced by a radical group. Each one of us has our own mental mapping. Most of us do not have such extreme beliefs, therefore our actions and experiences in life are vastly different.

What we feed ourselves can become our reality. They say you are what you eat. If you are feeding yourself good, positive messages, then you'll find yourself in a more positive world. If you are feeding yourself evil, negative messages, then you'll find yourself adapting to that world.

I say often, *are you happening to life, or is life happening to you?*

What I mean is, are you in control of your thoughts or does life determine them for you? Are you coasting through life without the awareness that you have a say in what you are thinking, how you are feeling, how you react?

To change your thoughts, you first need to recognize them. Then, understand what belief is supporting that thought. When you change your belief then your response will change.   You can now control if you get angry, scared, anxious, afraid, mad, happy, anything! Controlling the thought at the root and telling it where to go will help you remap your neuroplasticity (the path) if you have thoughts and reactions that don't serve you.

The brain controls thought, emotion, touch, breathing, memory, motor skill, vision, breathing, and hunger- so this three-pound organ is critical to protect! You are the only one that is responsible for your thoughts, your beliefs, and your actions. Believe it or not, this is the only thing you can actually control.

Mind

Whereas the brain is an organ, the mind is the manifestation of thoughts, perceptions, emotions, determination, imagination, and memory that occurs within the brain. The brain is the physical control center, but the mind is the experiences that happen with the data that goes into the center. The mind is using data from the brain to create an experience. The brain then responds to what the mind created.

Think of scrabble. There are a bunch of letters in a pile and you start to pick up pieces and create words. The scrambled letters you pick up are just pieces; they're data. They don't mean anything until you start to form words. Then you put the letters back on to the board and you get a certain number of points based on where you put the letters. The mind has a perception or thought of how the letters should be used and they lay them down on the board. This is the mind to brain relationship. The brain is the scrambled letters and the board. Once you have those letters in place then your board is created and you build off of what you've laid down (the paths you created as we discussed earlier).

The mind is energy. It thinks, feels, and chooses. Once it chooses, then it tells the brain what to do. The mind came up with the word and determined where it would go. When you put the pieces down, the brain had a path, a direction. The mind and the brain have two different functions, yet they are inseparable; they have a symbiotic relationship.

When you are able to control and manage your mind (perception, emotion, imagination), then you're able to have better control over the response your brain produces. This comes in the form of anger, fear, resentment, confidence. We can control these responses if we get a handle on the mind.

Mindset

Mindset is how we set our mind. It's the channel we tune our mental radio station to. The mind is the place where you have your thoughts, and the mindset is the general attitude you have. You can choose to tune your station to static (negativity) or you can choose a station where you hear the music clearly (positivity). This is entirely your call. You get to turn the dial on where you want your mindset to be; negative or positive, happy or mad, anxious or calm.

If you want a positive mindset, then you're telling your mind that you want positive thoughts, emotions, and perceptions. Happiness, positivity, confidence, peace are all mindsets, they're all attitudes.

"Whether you think you can or you can't, you're right," Henry Ford.

If you believe you can do something, then you can. If you tell yourself you can't, then you can't. This is your general attitude toward the situation, and you have full control over how you choose to perceive your reality.

I had a client tell me she needed to be anxious because she had to be able to provide for her kids. What her belief system told her was that she couldn't provide for her kids without being in a state of anxiety. When we dissected her belief system, she disclosed that her parents were always anxious when she was growing up until she got out of college. At this point, they were able to relax because their financial obligation was complete. Therefore, she believed that in order to get her kids through college, she would only be successful if she was anxious. Anxiety equated to results in her belief system.

I then asked her if it was possible for someone to make

money without being anxious. She said, "yes." I then asked her if when she's anxious if she performs at her highest level. She said, "no." I then asked her if she believes if *anxiety equaled results* or *results equaled results*.

She could see the limitations within her belief system. She even went on to say that when she's anxious she often sabotages herself. She finds herself crippled with pressure and it takes her longer to get her job done. Since her salary was commission based, the time-to-fill directly impacted her paycheck. I could see a lightbulb come on that her belief system was holding her back and counterproductive to what she was set on accomplishing.

She needed to have more trust and belief in herself. She needed to believe the world was working for her. She needed to have a more positive outlook on life. When she made that decision to have a different mindset then her mind saw different options. It then told the brain what new path to take. All three work in tandem.

You are in control of the decision-making process if you realize you have a choice. This took me 35-years to figure out, so if your lightbulb just went off—welcome to the party.

Like the woman in the example here, it never occurred to her that the way to break out of her anxiety was to change her mindset and her belief system. In order to do that, all she needed to do was make a new choice. I asked what new decision would serve her and she decided that anxiety does not equal results and it limits her potential. She also said that being in a state of peace and flow will yield better results to allow her to make more money.

Boom! YES! And that's exactly what she did! Then, whenever the old belief system would crop up, she would walk herself through the decision matrix and she would find herself in a state of peace, not anxiety. Does this way of thinking serve me?

Mindset takes work; this isn't a one-and-done. This is something that is going to come up and challenge you every day- especially when it comes to confidence.

Bear with me, we're almost done. I know this is a lot, but I'd encourage you to not glaze over these sections, but to really process what's being said.

Confidence and Mindset

Confidence is a mindset. It's the radio frequency we set our mind to, which then impacts the mind, and ultimately lays the pathways in the brain to tell our motor skills how to respond. If your brain isn't wired to be confident now, be intentional and tell it what you choose. Then, it's getting control of your thoughts and perceptions. If your beliefs are incongruent with the mindset you want to have, then your beliefs don't serve you and you need to change them.

When you get this level of control, then you can remap and train your brain to be more confident. It will start to become more natural for you, almost on auto-pilot.

Confidence is not something you can buy on a shelf. It's your attitude toward what you're doing, your attitude toward life. It's a series of choices and decisions you make that impact your beliefs about yourself. Confidence is having trust, faith, and belief in yourself, and this is narrative you need to start believing.

I want you to feel confident every day. It's not hard, but it's work. Commit right now to believing that you too can do this; I know you can.

Oh, and if you don't wear a helmet when you're riding a motorcycle, please consider it. That's your command center you've got up there and it has a big responsibility!

That's it for the technical part, but it's important. Thanks for sticking with me!

One last time to drill it in:

"Whether you think you can or you can't, you're right."

-Henry Ford

Chapter 6: Is an Imposter in You?

"What if they find out I've never been a manager before?"

"What if they find out I'm only 30-years-old, will they take me seriously?"

"What if I screw up?"

"What if my employees don't take me seriously and they overthrow me?"

Goodness, I remember the first time I had employees reporting to me. It was terrifying. I was a young manager, at least compared to my peers. I was working in information technology, a male-dominated industry, and I always felt I had to prove myself at 140% to be taken seriously.

Not only was I a female, but I was young. I wanted to

show my boss he could trust me, he could have faith in me, that I was capable of doing the job that he hired me for. But I was also scared out my mind.

On my 30th birthday, my parents flew to California, where I was living, and I'll never forget their little adventure into the office. I was sitting in a meeting that I was conducting, and I looked over to see some commotion at the door. A Vice President walked in the room, followed then by the admin, some other coworkers, and then….my parents.

They barged in the room singing *Happy Birthday* and holding flowers and a cake that said *Happy 30th Birthday* right in the center of the cake. This was my worst fear staring right back at me. I didn't want anyone to know how old I was and now it was being presented to the entire office in the form of a cake!

I quickly saw that the number 30 was written on a clear piece of plastic and without any hesitation, I grabbed that piece of plastic and licked it before anyone else could see how old I actually was.

It was my imposter syndrome staring at me in the face. It was everything I tried to hide because I didn't think I'd be taken seriously if they knew just how young I was. I panicked. I was in fear. I was about to be outted to the entire office….and then what? This was bad. This was really bad.

At least that's how I saw it.

If you've not heard of imposter syndrome, there's a high probability you've dealt with it at some point in your life. It's believing that you are not good enough, smart enough, worthy enough to take on a task, and 70% of people deal with this during their lifetime! God forbid anyone finds out, it could be detrimental!

Maybe you've found yourself saying:

- I'm a fraud
- Someone else should be doing this
- I'm not good enough
- Will they find out that I'm not qualified?
- Will they believe me?
- How will they take me seriously?
- Will they give the task to someone else when they find out the truth?
- They're on to me!

Quite painful, actually. It's like hiding a secret inside of you and just waiting for yourself to slip up once and then the world will crumble around you. At least, that's what it feels like, but it doesn't mean that's actually going to happen.

Confidence and imposter syndrome do not play in the same space, in fact, they are counter to each other.

One says, *I got this no matter what*, where the other says *I'm one step away from everything falling apart!* Two completely different energies and mindsets.

Imposter syndrome has been tied to perfectionism, where we have a belief that, in order to be responsible to execute on something, we have to be perfect at it. This gives us very little room to grow and expand into a role; we should already possess the skills before taking on the task or the role.

I don't know about you, but I don't know one person that started out with experience and knowing how to do everything. Think about a person you respect for their leadership or a company they built. Have you looked at their resume? I'll bet they weren't a CEO at 16 years of age! We all had to start with our first job, mediocre salary, and even our first experience as a manager. You don't go from zero to sixty, but imposter syndrome has you believing you need to have it all in order to be taken seriously.

This is a pressure you put on yourself and it can be crippling. That dirty secret you hold on to that is always so close to being exposed. You do everything you can to keep it locked away, but it's there, pushing on the door, and it's a matter of time until it gets out.

Let's go back to the impromptu birthday part.

This terrifying situation where my parents came bursting into a meeting that I was conducting to sing me happy birthday and to announce to the office that I was a child. Mortifying!

Or was it?

It was mortifying, at the time. But that's the power of the mind.

Took me years to break past this imposter syndrome, change my mindset, and gain confidence in myself to understand that this was one of the kindest and sweetest gestures my parents could have done, but my imposter syndrome killed the moment.

> My parents flew all the way across the country, from Virginia, to be with me on my 30th birthday since I was alone. I couldn't take a day off work because I needed to be a good employee and show up six-days a week to prove myself.
>
> On my birthday, my parents came into the office with a cake and flowers to surprise me. They figured out how to get in the building, who could bring them to me, and they came in with all their love and excitement to surprise me.
>
> And me...I was mortified.
>
> The entire office was going to know how old I was. Would my team take me seriously? Would my peers take me seriously? Would people look at me differently?
>
> How was I going to recover from this?

My fear, my anxiety, my lack of confidence trumped the beauty of this kind gesture.

I didn't have to go into panic mode. The office wasn't going to collapse because of this birthday situation. My team wasn't going to overthrow me. My life wasn't going to be over if people knew I was 30 years old. That was the imposter living within me.

The situation very well could have played out like this:

> My two loving parents flew to California to be with me on my 30th birthday. I didn't know anyone in California, and they didn't want me to spend my birthday alone. While I was at work, they found out where to buy a cake and they had it customized just for me. They picked up the cake, bought a bouquet of pink and yellow flowers, and came to surprise their first born at work for this big milestone birthday.

> They figured out how to get in the building, who could bring them to me, and they came in with all their love and excitement to surprise me.

> I looked over and saw the two wonderful humans that gave me life and raised me. Here I was, working in the office on my birthday and truly, I just wanted to be hanging out with them! I was so excited to see them, it was exactly what I needed! I had no idea they were coming, and I love surprises! I'm usually the one giving surprises, rarely the one getting surprises, and this was so amazing that would

do all of this for me!

My office loved the cake, it was a nice thing to share with everyone. I had only been working there a few months, so it gave some people an opportunity to come wish me happy birthday that hadn't had a chance to meet me yet.

This was such an unforgettable birthday and I'm grateful for such amazing humans to love me and be there for me.

I wish I could honestly say the latter was my initial experience, but it is how I view the situation now. There's no difference as to the events that took place in these situations, only in the perception. Imposter syndrome will create all kinds of uncertainty and unnecessary suffering.

Imagine a world where we always saw the latter. Where it didn't matter how old we were. Where it didn't matter if you didn't have all the skills. Where you were OK with learning as you went through life instead of needing to know everything up front. That can be your reality. Confidence will push aside that imposter when you tell yourself that everything will be OK no matter what. It's a mindset.

Confidence is a mindset and a choice you make. The world can be for you, or it can be against you. You can believe that you have everything you need inside of you, or you can be in fear of what you believe you don't have. You can trust that everything is going to work out, or you can choose to believe that your world is going to come crashing down in an instance. Only you choose the mindset to your reality.

My dad always said that his career in the navy was like being thrown into one new job assignment after another, for which he was totally inexperienced and unqualified. He had to come up to speed and succeed quickly or fail. Sink or swim he called it. He went from working on a submarine to running a grocery store to managing financial software systems. Very often, my dad had very little experience in the next job he was assigned to. Allowing the imposter to thrive would have been a sure career killer. If he had allowed himself to be held back because of fear, because he didn't feel qualified enough, because he didn't feel skilled enough, then his career would have taken a very different path. The reason my dad was able to continue to climb the ranks was because he faced everything he was given and learned how to do it!

One thing about my dad is he has always been able to figure anything out. It doesn't matter if it was doing electrical, building a theater, making shelves, or growing a vineyard, nothing has been unsurmountable for my father. Whereas factually, he may not know how to do something, he has always known that he'll be able to figure it out (and he knows when to ask for help- most times, anyhow).

My dad has developed a trust within himself that he can do new things. It's impressive to watch him go into action and start to research. I've watched this my entire life and it has absolutely impacted my *can do* attitude. What I've learned from my dad is that you can do anything. If you allow an imposter to thrive within you then you'll miss lots of opportunities in life.

As a leader, you aren't expected to know everything. You're expected to get the job done. Know what you're good at, where you need expert advice, and who to surround yourself with to help you get the job done. Don't put the pressure on yourself that *YOU* have to know it all, you just need to get it done. If you're willing to learn, willing to ask for help, willing to leave your ego at the door, then you're well ahead of people that get paralyzed when they're faced with something they don't know how to do.

If there's an imposter inside of you, that voice will go away when you learn to trust and believe in yourself. The trick is to understand the voice of the imposter so you can tell it that it's all going to be OK.

In order to get rid of negative feelings, I used to suppress them. What I've found far more effective is to face them.

Your reactions are a window to what's happening on the inside. When you react, when you feel something, that's a glimpse at what you believe. When your mind is telling you that you're not good enough, smart enough, that you're a fraud- that should indicate an opportunity for you. Same is true with any state of suffering; fear, frustration, anger, resentment, anxiety, boredom, embarrassment, and anything that doesn't make you feel good. This should be an opportunity for you to ask yourself why you don't feel good enough. Why you don't feel qualified enough. Why you don't feel smart enough, pretty enough, strong enough. Then face these thoughts, acknowledge them, and assure yourself that you are all those thing. Affirm yourself!

There is a purpose for pain. If you didn't feel pain, then it could be dangerous if you stepped on a nail or put your hand on a hot stove. Pain is designed to get your attention. Once you see it, then it's up to you to address it appropriately. Use it for what it's designed for and take control of the situation.

I like to ask myself this question; Does this serve me?

If you learn to ask yourself those simple four words, then you'll find some powerful answers that will change the way you show up in the world. You'll be able to navigate any situation to find the life you want to create. If it's a negative situation then it's probably not serving you. Does negative energy help you in life? Do you sleep better when you have negativity inside of you? Do you have clarity of thoughts with negativity? Think through all the scenarios to help you find your true truth.

As you stretch yourself into new levels of yourself, you may feel like an imposter. If you've done something a million times, you don't typically question if you can do the thing. It's like driving. After you've done it enough, you just drive, you don't worry about changing lanes and avoiding highways. You might not even remember the drive because you're so familiar with the route and the process.

This imposter will come into play when you've stepped into new territories, new heights, new goals, bigger dreams. It's not there to hurt you, only to keep you safe. It doesn't know the new world, so sometimes it tells you to go back to what it already knows, what it's familiar with, where it feels safe. You are in control of that voice, and the first step is to recognize and maybe even thank the voice.

It's like your grandma telling you not to skydive out of an airplane because she doesn't want you to get hurt. Kindly thank her for the concern. Tell her it's going to be OK. Then go do the jump and experience the feeling of the wind in your hair. When you're done, go thank your grandma for her concern and let her know you're fine.

Go get your parachute to jump out of the plane and into living this life. Tell yourself that you're going to be OK and enjoy the experience. No one said that growth would be comfortable, it won't be, but it's necessary to get to that next level of you. Know that you don't have to be the one to know it all, you can ask for help along the way! No one expects you to know everything, so consult with experts to help you figure out whatever task you're solving. Most importantly, trust yourself. Trust that you'll get through it, you'll figure it out, and everything will be OK. Ask yourself *does this serve me?* If it doesn't then figure out a more powerful belief (we'll dig into beliefs here in a bit).

At the end of the day, confidence is a mindset. You have it inside of you and all you need to do is train the six inches between your ears to work for you and not against you.

"Live from the heart of yourself. Seek to be whole, not perfect."

— Oprah Winfrey

Chapter 7: You Choose Your Experience

You always have a choice if you know you have one, but you can't fight a battle if you don't know you're in one.

When I ask if you are happening to life or if life is happening to you, it comes down to choice. If you are in a place of suffering, then life is happening to you. It means that you have given up your choice on how you want to feel (grieving excluded). Most people don't realize they have an option in their happiness, their success, how they show up, their confidence—life chooses for them.

There isn't one person I've met that would choose to be, let's say, angry over being happy. Yet, we often find ourselves angered and frustrated. Someone does wrong by you. Someone cuts you off on the road.

Someone steals something from you. It's frustrating, no doubt, but you have the choice not to get angry.

It goes back to the powerful question you should be asking yourself; does this serve me? Does it serve me to feel this way? Most of the time, NO. You don't have clarity of mind when you're angry. You don't have clarity of mind when you're in any state of suffering. You get so focused on the negative emotion and it consumes you.

Anger is one of the many states of suffering we can involuntarily find ourselves in. Likely, none of these you would consciously choose to feel:

- Fearful
- Frustrated
- Angry
- Resentful
- Anxious
- Bored
- Embarrassed
- Lonely
- Afraid
- Annoyed
- Nervous
- Tense
- Alarmed

Given the choice, you'd rather be:

- Excited
- Happy
- Amused
- Calm
- Relaxed
- Satisfied
- Content
- Peaceful
- Loved
- Joyful
- Fulfilled
- Confident

If you don't realize you have a choice, then your mind will default to what it knows. What it knows doesn't always mean it will serve you best.

Having a choice mindset will allow you to have options in your life. It will give you the power to decide how you want to feel, show up, or be in any situation. A choice mindset doesn't see glass ceilings and caged walls. Rather, it sees limitless options and unlimited potential. It's a growth mindset versus a fixed mindset.

Your choices are limitless when you allow your mind to expand. Life is far more than your first reaction. Mindset is an art and it's a choice. You have to tell your brain where to go. Lead it, don't allow it to lead you.

The life you want is between your two ears. It's far too easy to get into a negative space, not believe in yourself, have thoughts that don't serve you. When you do, you're giving your brain a command to find justifications. It's like a Google search. Whatever command you put in the *search* will spit out a result. Remember, *garbage in, garbage out!* The idea is to catch your thoughts in real time so you can divert them.

Tony Robbins says, "Where your thoughts go, your energy flows." If you choose to be positive, you'll find reasons to support your thoughts. If you give in to suffering, you'll find reasons to support those thoughts.

When suffering arises, acknowledge the thinking and tell your brain where it should go. Tell yourself that you trust in your abilities, that you have faith the world is working for you, that it will be OK no matter what the outcome. Point your thoughts to confident thoughts and that's what search result your brain will produce.

But what choice did you have about getting laid off?

Well, you chose to work for a company, and they have the right to downsize. You can also choose to look at it as an opportunity! Maybe it's time to change industries, or build a business, find a new job all together, or maybe even retire. There are lots of choices when you open your mind and look for them.

How many times have you heard someone losing their job and they end up finding a better company, making more money, or find more happiness? When unexpected things happen, your brain may take you to a dark place. It's your job catch these thoughts and take them to a more secure and trusting place.

There are always choices you have. You can choose:

- To let go
- To hold on
- To believe
- To accept
- To move forward
- To stop
- To want better
- To want more
- To want less
- To accept what you have
- To be happy
- To be miserable (read that again- because yes, it's a choice you make!)
- To ask for help
- To do it alone
- To not look for lessons
- To take accountability
- To blame
- To be who you are
- To be someone else
- To be uncomfortable
- Over your perception
- Over your actions
- Over your emotions
- Who you hang out with
- Over what you listen to
- Over your thoughts

You get to choose if you want to be confident. If you want to believe in yourself and place trust in yourself.

Even in situations that seem dark and optionless, you will always have options. If you don't see them, then that's how you've chosen to look at the situation; one dimensional.

While under the David Bayer Coaching program, it was ingrained in me that the brain is a goal achieving machine. Whatever you put your mind to becomes your reality. If you think you can, you can. If you think you can't, you can't. Whichever direction you choose, you'll start finding justifications for why that is true. If you're a failure, you'll find reasons to believe that. If you're a winner, you'll find justifications to substantiate that. Your brain wants goals. Your thoughts are your goals. You're the master and whatever thoughts you choose your brain wants to find reasons and justifications to support them. This is why it's important to make sure your thoughts align with how you want to live and who you want to be.

~~~

I had a friend message me recently and asked this question. "What is the root of fear and anxiety? How can you squash it?"

My answer, "Beliefs. Change your beliefs."

When you peel back the source of your anxiety, stress,

and states of suffering, you'll find your belief system at the core. Beliefs are ideas that you hold as true and correct.

Imagine you lose your hearing. You once heard the world around you and now you're Deaf. You never thought about hearing because it was always there. You didn't realize how most everything you do is integrated with hearing. Your alarm clock, your music, the ice maker, knowing when someone's coming in the door, when a text message comes through, even hearing the upstairs neighbors when they get home from work. There were sounds in everything about your life, now that's all gone. What about concerts, talking on the phone with your best friend, what about Facetiming with your niece? What's going to happen to your job in sales? What will happen to your relationship with the new person you're dating? What will driving be like when an ambulance comes up behind you? What will the holiday caroling with the family be like? What about talking with your friends? Life, it's just not the same.

How would you respond?

There may be some tears now that you've lost your hearing. It's kind of scary to enter this unknown world you just ventured into. You've seen Deaf people living happy lives, but that's them! Those Deaf people didn't have your life in a hearing world, so it's different. I don't doubt that you also feel a level of discomfort in this new norm.

You believe your life is over. You believe nothing will ever be the same. You believe your partner will leave you. You believe it's hard to be Deaf.

These are all choices you can make to believe, but do they serve you?

What if you told yourself that being Deaf is no different than hearing? In fact, you know that you'll have other senses that will be heightened because you can no longer hear. What if you believed that your partner and friends would stick with you no matter what (and if they didn't then they weren't good friends in the first place)? What if you believed this was part of the design for your life and you were going to embrace it with open arms? How different would your world look if you addressed your beliefs?

If you change your beliefs, then your brain will start to validate your thoughts.

Ludwig van Beethoven, born in Germany in 1770, is one of the most well-known composers and pianists. He's revered as one of the most talented classical music composers that ever lived. In 1800, he shared his first renowned piece of work, "First Symphony," and composed many famous works of art over the next 27 years before his death. Ludwig was known for pieces such as "Turkish March," 'Missa Solemnis," and "Last Piano Concerto." If you've not had the opportunity to listen to Beethoven's masterpieces, it's truly a remarkable experience.

Before the release of Ludwig's first piece of music in 1800, he started to lose his hearing, and over the course of his life he went completely deaf.

Imagine. You're a famous composer. You've studied. You've practiced. You've spent your entire life dedicated to learning and crafting a musical talent to share with the world and you lose your hearing. Imagine what that would be like.

I can imagine the frustration of losing your hearing as a composer, but it didn't stop Ludwig. He found other ways to stay in tune with the music; through his other senses. Ludwig believed he could still be great, and he was. Ludwig believed in his skills, his mission, himself. Although his hearing went away, it didn't stop him because he believed he was bigger than the problem.

Beliefs are created from experiences or input from others. They impact your experiences. If you were bit by a dog, you may have an opinion that dogs are scary. Now, when you see a dog, you go into a state of fear. Your current experience is impacted by your past experiences. If you change your belief that not all dogs are scary then you can change your experience.

People often mistake beliefs and facts.

Facts are tangible.

- You need air to breathe
- You will die one day
- It takes a sperm and an egg to make a baby
- George Washington was the first US President
- Kamala Harris was the first female US Vice President
- The largest state in the United States is Alaska
- The smallest state in the United States in Rhode Island

Beliefs vary from person to person.

- My dad is a great cook
- My mom is a saint
- The apple is delicious
- My presence is needed
- Life can't go on without him
- People should wear clothes to cover their shoulders in the office
- My cat is the sweetest
- Snakes are scary
- The movie was funny
- That person looks sad

Beliefs form your reality, but they do not necessarily have to be factual. I believe my dad is a great cook, but someone that doesn't enjoy the kind of food he makes may think differently. I believe apples are delicious, but you may hate the taste. We are all right because they're beliefs, not facts. There is no right and no wrong, it's what is true to each one of us. We can have different beliefs and both be correct, but facts have only one truth. Two plus two equals four, that's fact.

Because beliefs are created in your mind and not fact, the key is to understand the difference and know what you can control.

My entire life I've had people comment about my height. I believed these comments were rude and meant to harm me, at least this is the way I thought when I was younger. Nowadays, I hear the same comments and they don't phase me.

What changed?

I changed my beliefs. I exercised the power of a choice mindset. I understood what I could control and what I couldn't. I couldn't control how tall I was, but I could control my beliefs. I made the choice to believe that I was made perfect. I made the choice to believe my body was designed just for me. I chose to believe that only I was responsible for my happiness. I chose to believe that not everyone was against me. I chose to believe that people are good, and inquisitive, and that many people are just insecure and jealous.

My prior beliefs were causing me to go into a state of suffering and they weren't serving me. I made the decision to change my thinking. It came down to a change in my beliefs. I was not a victim; I made that choice to stop believe I was. When I did, the way I experienced life started to serve me.

I was sitting in a bar in Germany with my friend, Brittany, when I was 20, and the bartender took a liking to us. We didn't speak German, and he didn't speak English. Through smiles, sign language, and alcohol we managed to somehow communicate. This man was probably about 60 years of age. He was shorter in stature and had thick, white hair. He was enamored by me. We didn't speak the same language, but he enjoyed talking to me, that was clear!

At some point, he disappeared.

I didn't think much of it, I was busy talking with Brittany and enjoying our first trip to Germany! From out of nowhere, the little bartender reappeared. He brought with him a ladder. He plunked the ladder down next to me and confidently walked up to the fourth rung. He looked down and me and with his hand he gestured me to stand up. And then...I knew. I knew what was coming next. I stood up, and no sooner than I had fully stood in an upright position, my bartender friend was giving me a big bear hug.

We all laughed! There were 3 people at the other end of the bar (no one spoke English) and we all shared in laughter and then came another round of shots from the bartender.

I'll never forget that moment. I don't know one person in my life that has ever had anything remotely close to that happen to them.

Only me.

I remember a time when I was standing next to a building in Italy talking on the phone. As I was chatting, I saw someone running on the same block as me. The boy was fast, Roadrunner fast. He whizzed past me and I remember thinking he probably had some place very important to go. As he passed me, he looked over and he immediately stopped. Apparently, he hadn't seen me up until that very moment. It felt like I was watching a cartoon where the Roadrunner was running past me. In the moment he saw me, he stopped. *BING* (was the sound I heard in my head). Just like the cartoon. He took two steps back towards me and said, "Quanto sei alta?" Which means, *how tall are you*? I replied "186 centimetri" (six foot, one inch).

Roadrunner processed the data in half a second, said "OK," and then he kept running!

Unique interaction, for sure.

I was in a 7-Eleven in Arizona once and a little girl spotted me as I was picking out my beef jerky. She pointed at me, looked at her mother and said, "Mommy, she's so high!" Her mom looked at me and said, "Honey, she's not high, she's very tall!" They then broke out in some bizarre duo of a song that I'm guessing they made up. I'll never forget the words or the tune, "she is so tall, she is so beautiful, she is so tall, she is so beautiful….," and on and on and on. They didn't stop. It's like their record player broke and they kept singing! I didn't have an issue with being called tall or beautiful, per sey, but it was a little random and weird to have a mother/daughter duo clearly singing about me in this pitstop in the middle of Arizona. True story, no embellishing.

As I reflected on all these interesting situations in my life, I made the choice to believe they were unique blessing. They were colorful. They were fun. People were finding ladders to hug me. Roadrunner was caught midstream and stopped so he could ask me a question. A woman and her daughter invented a song and sang it publicly on my behalf. I could have believed people were making fun of me, but I chose differently. I started to experience life fuller when I made the powerful decisions to change my beliefs about myself and accept who I am.

Beliefs are powerful. They can serve you or they can limit you.

Remember my client who thought she needed to be anxious in order to make money? When she realized that was neither fact nor truth, she changed her belief system. When she did, she was able find more clarity and peace (and she actually ended up making more money).

She had a limiting belief system. Because she believed she needed to be anxious to make money, she robbed herself of joy, peace, and happiness. As soon as she changed her belief, then she was able to experience life more abundantly (and a more abundant bank account).

When you start to understand that beliefs are at the core of all your experiences, then if you want a different experience you need to change your beliefs.

How many times have you looked at a situation and thought it was too complicated to figure out?

How many times have you wanted to do something, but you didn't know where to start so you didn't?

How many times have you been too afraid to attempt something because of the fear of the unknown?

Tapping into your confidence and having confident beliefs are going to help you smash whatever is holding you back. Tell your brain where to go. Again, don't let it lead you, you take charge.

Here's some examples of how to change your internal dialogue to a more confident mindset.

Old Limiting Belief	New Belief
I can't do something that is complicated	I can figure anything out I put my mind to
People will judge you if you fail	People will respect me for trying
I have to figure it all out on your own	People will help me get to where I want to be
The unknown is scary	The unknown is exciting
Discomfort is uncomfortable	Discomfort symbolizes growth
People will laugh at me for being different	People will embrace me for being unique

By merely changing your beliefs then you are able to change your entire experience. You are able to open yourself up to more possibilities and the way you show up in this world.

We know confidence is a mindset and mindset is a belief system. If you believe you can't do something, then you can't. If you believe that anything is possible, then anything is possible. Your beliefs are more than just believing if aliens exist or not. Beliefs drive possibility, experiences, happiness, confidence.

When I made the decision I was going to go public with my personal story, it was one of the most scary and liberating decisions I ever made. It was like this weight came off me and I could finally breathe. It was an evolution as I inched my way forward to telling my story. At first, I thought there was absolutely no way I was going to be able to let people know the truth. I would surely ruin my career and people would disassociate themselves with me.

Then, I started to put myself in the shoes of people that needed to hear my story. I came to the conclusion that I needed to get my story out into the world for their sake. But I should use an alias? I can come out with my story, but I won't use my name.

Then I dug deeper within myself and listened to what my gut was telling me. My story needed to come out with my name. If my company was going to let me go, then was that the kind of company I really wanted to work for? And, if people weren't going to support me, were they the kinds of people I wanted in my life anyhow? I chose authenticity.

I changed how I viewed the situation. I went from scared to empowered. I went from wondering what would happen to being more curious about what impact would be missed if I didn't come forward. My confidence grew because I took my limiting beliefs and changed them around to empower myself instead. The millimeter shifts took me from being nervous to owner of my destiny. I didn't have to change as a person, I just needed to change my beliefs and that changed the experience. I could walk forward with ease.

I remember getting my first adverse response to sharing my story.

"Jen, you should be ashamed of yourself putting your message out there and subjecting others to it."

I'm not going to lie, that stung. But I also knew where it was coming from. This was from a guy that was so wrapped up in drugs, his family disowned him, and he couldn't break free from the madness of his world. He was probably high when he wrote the message, may have been jealous or envious, I have no idea. I knew a lot of his journey and it was a rocky one.

Shrapnel. It was just shrapnel. I was caught in his line of fire driven by his beliefs. Just because he believed that I shouldn't be sharing my story didn't mean I needed to be of the same belief. Just because he thought I was polluting the world didn't mean I was. In fact, I had received a lot of amazing feedback on how my story had helped people gain strength, so clearly, he was spouting an opinion and not a fact.

It's easy to get wrapped up in your own limiting beliefs or other people's opinions and beliefs. When you feel dissonance within yourself, peel back the onion and ask yourself what beliefs are causing you to feel the way you do. And, back to the most powerful question you can ask yourself, does that way of thinking serve you? If the answer is NO, then it's a limiting belief. It's limiting you from your right to thrive.

Take control over your choices and your beliefs. Your glass is half-full *OR* it is half-empty (or you can be like my friend, Dean, who says "I'm just happy to have anything in my cup at all!"). Believe how you want your life to look and your brain will find the possibilities to support them.

Life is going to throw things at you that you don't expect or think is fair. You may even get blindsided and your confidence gets shaken. Just when you think you've got a solid footing within yourself, you may find a limiting belief hidden somewhere that starts to hold you back. It's having a constant connection with yourself and being able to identify what you control and don't control that will help you stay on the course.

We all live. We all die. We all breathe. We all blink. Our hearts beat. Our lungs take in air. The mind is what sets you apart (and sure, we physically look different). You control how you think. You can confidently show up in the world and have the life you want if you lead your mind there. Be the leader. Happen to life. And know that you always have a choice and your beliefs drive your experiences.

Choice is power.

Beliefs are powerful.

Confidence is queen.

Knowledge is power, and now you know.

"We are all in the gutter, but some of us are looking at the stars."

-Oscar Wilde

.

Chapter 8: Knowing Your WHY

Have you ever stopped to ask yourself what your purpose is in life? If someone asked you your purpose, what would you say? Purpose gives meaning to life. It's more than passion, which is what you like to do, but rather the reason for your existence. Purpose gives you a motive to get out of bed. It gives you reason to go out and face the day. Without meaning why would anything matter? When you live a purposeful life and are connected to your *why* then you elevate your confidence. Goal striving and achieving enhances self-confidence. It helps you not only define who you are and gives identity, but it's also the spark to propel you forward and can bring immense gratification.

I think of my niece, Olive, and at two-years-old, her purpose is to be happy and play with her toys! She doesn't go to school, doesn't pay the bills, she isn't building the company of her dreams…..yet. Today, she's all about playing with her bear, Snuggles! The bear brings her so much joy, she can't wait to get up to go drag him around the house with her! Oh, and pancakes. I'm pretty sure her purpose is to eat pancakes too! One day, she'll grow up and her purpose will change, all the way until she reaches her very old age. Whatever her reason, I hope she always has some motive to get out of bed.

I've not seen Olive get up for the day and question what she should do. She's focused on being happy. If she's not, she'll let you know. I've not seen her aimlessly walk around wondering what to do, she's always finding something to keep her entertained and make her happy. That's her purpose! As adults, playing with toys may be more of a passion, but if you can find a way to turn that into purpose then more power to you!

If we don't have purpose, what are we driving towards? What keeps us going? What keeps us from giving up?

Have you heard about people that pass away after they retire? They haven't found another purpose and their zest for life changes.

I've told this story before, but it makes me laugh every time I think about it.

I went on a date one time with a guy that came from a lineage of money. We didn't have any in-depth conversation before we met, our pizza date was our first real conversation (side note, he ate before we met so it was odd from the start).

I will never forget asking him about what he does.

"So, what do you do?"

"Nothing."

"Oh, OK." [in my head I'm thinking- maybe a better question to ask *before* the date.]

"I come from money, so I don't have to do anything."

"Oh, OK." [huge turn off, should I run?] "That's interesting, do you have any goals, any hobbies?"

"No. Not really. Well, it's to get out of bed every day and not spend all my money."

My mind was *BLOWN*! I'm someone that is goal oriented and structured, I couldn't imagine not having anything that I was working towards! I workout so I can feel good and stay in shape. I work so I can pay my bills and retire one day. I make time for friends so I can have social interaction in my life. I go to church so I can have communion with others and sing praises. I have loads of things that give me purpose and this guy was striving to get out of bed?!

I was in shock. I don't have anyone in my life that fits this mold of having no purpose and I was ready to run. I was also fascinated by this alien and I wanted to know more! This guy had to force himself out of the bed, that was his goal! He didn't aim to feel good, be a contributing member of society, volunteer, change the world. NO! He merely wanted to get out of bed. I most certainly started asking the question of purpose before any dates going forward, this was a non-starter for me. But I was fascinated in the moment listening to this meaningless babble as ate pizza by myself.

Purpose gets you out of bed. Purpose is motivation. Purpose will help give you confidence. Purpose is the reason you were born. Purpose will give you the strength to push down any obstacle that gets in the way of what you're designed to do.

Purpose gives you your *why*.

If you don't know, ask yourself some of these questions:

- What regret not doing later in your life?
- What makes you feel good?
- What are you good at?
- What do people ask you to do?
- What are your dreams and aspirations?
- What does your perfect world look like?
- What impact do you want to have on this world?
- What do you want to be remembered for?
- Who do you want to help in this world?

Don't put limits on your answers, allow your mind to dream, to see, to envision. You are a vessel and the world works through you. If you woke up today, there's a reason, a purpose, a *why* you're still here. What is that for you without limitations?

It sounded crazy for a regular person to go to space, and yet Richard Branson was the first non-astronaut to go on July 11, 2021. While in space, he recorded a video:

> *"To all you kids down there, I was once a child with a dream looking up to the stars. Now, I'm an adult in a spaceship with lots of other wonderful adults looking down to our beautiful, beautiful earth. To the next generation of dreamers, if we can do this, just imagine what you can do"*

> -Richard Branson

Richard didn't put a cap on his imagination, his dream, his purpose. If we all thought it was an impossible dream, then none of us would go into space. Richard believed and he made it happen.

Imagine if Alexander Graham Bell didn't believe the telephone could exist, would we be talking on a phone today?

What about if Thomas Edison hadn't imagined the light bulb, would we all be restricted to seeing by sunlight or candlelight?

What if Louis Pasteur and Robert Koch didn't believe that antibiotics could actually be invented? Millions and millions of lives have been saved from this creation!

The list of possibilities is endless. Think of the inventions that have changed life as we know it.

- Computer
- Wheel
- Railroad
- Steel
- Refrigerator
- X-ray
- Concrete
- Fire
- Microwaves
- Television
- Camera
- Internet
- Email
- Credit Cards
- Robots
- Films
- Color TV

The list goes on and on. How different would life be if you limited yourself to believing only in what could be seen instead of allowing life to work through you for a grander design than even what you could imagine?

Don't get lost or overwhelmed in thinking you need to have a purpose that includes inventing a life-changing contraption. We don't have to compete with Richard Branson. Purpose can be raising children, spreading the word of God, rescuing animals, volunteering, building a business, being the best leader you can be, staying in gratitude and happiness. There is no single definition of purpose, it could be anything—if you allow your mind to experience limitless possibilities.

Let's say you're going to start training for a marathon. Maybe you've not done it before and you're more of a jogger than a runner. Would you expect that on day one of training that you go do your best 26-mile run? No, that's what training is for! With practice, you get a little better and you keep improving.

When we have purpose, we have a goal we are striving for. It doesn't mean that on day one we expect we are going to be perfect. It means that no matter what the obstacle, we have a mission to achieve and will get there by any means. Purpose is fuel to a fire. It helps ignite you from the inside out and makes you unstoppable. I think of my cat, Booger, when I put catnip in my hand. She knows there's something in there, and she won't stop until she gets what she wants. If I move rooms, she follows. If I close the door, she'll meow and try to break the door down. Her purpose becomes the treat, and nothing seems insurmountable because she's determined.

It's easy for us to get in our own heads and get stuck before we get started.

- What are people going to think?

- Other people are further along
- Am I going to look foolish?
- I don't know what I'm doing
- Am I going to be good enough?

Let me ask you this, would you laugh at a child taking their first step? No! We celebrate, we clap, we take videos and post them on social media! Yet, when it comes to ourselves, we become much more critical. What if you allowed yourself permission to grow? What if you met yourself where you were at and appreciated the steps and progress you made along the way?

When you know *why* you are doing something, you have determination, willpower, grit; just like when you started training for the marathon. You knew you weren't going to run your best race on day one (and quite frankly, you probably didn't do all 26.2 miles when you started). But you kept going. You kept practicing. You built your body up for the race. You continued to grow and stretch to new levels. Each new level you reach will require a new version of you. Fulfilling your purpose strengthens and enhances you, giving you more self-confidence in your skills and abilities.

Have you ever been walking on a sidewalk and suddenly, it's no longer flat? You trip on it because there's a break in the concrete and it's raised. Hopefully you're paying attention and don't fall, it seemed to come out of nowhere! Everything else was flat, where did this elevated bump come from?! It's most likely from the roots of a tree. Roots grow deep into the ground and they don't tend to care what's in their way. They can actually cause a lot of issues under the ground. You may have a sprinkler system, underground pipes, a driveway, a walkway, all of which the roots can impact. When you plant the tree, it doesn't have deep roots initially. As the tree grows into its full potential, the roots begin to grow and sprawl underneath the ground. The roots have a purpose. Their purpose is to anchor, support, store energy, and absorb water for the tree. It doesn't matter if there's a sidewalk, pipes, or a walkway, the roots have a very important job to complete. If it means breaking the sidewalk, then it breaks the sidewalk.

This is confidence.

The roots have trust, faith, belief in what they're doing and they'll go to any lengths to succeed. When you know what you are designed to do, when you know the mission you were put here for, when you know why you are doing what you are doing, then you are unstoppable. You have a fuel inside of you that will break any sidewalk in your path (metaphorically speaking).

If you had a child that fell in the pool and couldn't swim, wouldn't you do anything you could to save that child? Even if you couldn't swim, you would focus on your goal and get creative. You'd throw in a buoy, call someone over to help, or jump in anyway. Your purpose in that moment is to save the child. We can do amazing things when we set our mind to achieving a goal. It's like when you hear about someone flipping over a car to save someone trapped underneath. When you allow the purpose to flow through you, and you trust in the mission, then you can do anything.

Get quiet. Ask yourself the questions that help you to better understand what drives you. I want you to live intentionally. I don't want you to be blowing wherever the wind takes you, but rather those roots that know what they are made for and anchored with a purpose. You may have multiple purposes; you don't need to limit yourself to just one. They'll likely change over the course of your life, so always ask yourself why are you doing what you're doing. Are you speaking into the purpose that's designed for you? I suggest you get quiet and listen for the answers.

You can also think about purpose like a mission and vision statement.

Typical mission statements of a company outline what they want to achieve, who they support, and why. This is their purpose.

> **Southwest**: To be the world's most loved, most efficient, and most profitable airline.
>
> **Sweetgreen**: To inspire healthier communities by connecting people to real food.

Nordstrom: To give customers the most compelling shopping experience possible.

TED: Spread ideas.

Tesla: To accelerate the world's transition to sustainable energy.

Warby Parker: To offer designer eyewear at a revolutionary price, while leading the way for socially conscious businesses.

Then, you start to create the vision. The vision is how you want to execute on the mission.

You may be drawing a blank and that's OK. You might not have a specific mission statement in mind. Shoot for vaguer goals. Be happy. Be kind. Be at peace. Be healthy. Specific or vague, find your purpose. Have goals. Watch your confidence soar when you are connected to yourself and why you were brought on this earth.

Don't limit what you can do by what you can see. The world has already proven that humans can do miraculous things. You're here for a reason. If you woke up today, there's a purpose for you. Find it and let it fuel you. You are an unstoppable human being, and just like those roots, your purpose will have you doing amazing things. Confidence will flourish when you know why you're here.

"Don't ask yourself what the world needs, ask yourself what makes you come alive. And then go and do that. Because what the world needs is people who have come alive."

-Howard Washington Thurman

Chapter 9: Comparing: The Confidence Killer

The fastest way to kill or falsely elevate your confidence is to compare yourself to others.

Confidence isn't about walking into room and believing you're better than everyone. It also doesn't require you to be validated by anyone. Confidence is walking into a room and being secure with who you are regardless of who is there.

Confidence is like Solitaire. It doesn't require anyone else. Everything you need is inside of you. Period.

There's this strange phenomenon with being tall. People treat me like a human tape measure. They're always walking up and seeing how tall they are compared to me. It's honestly like I'm one of those measuring sticks when you were a kid to see if you were tall enough to ride the ride. I don't know why this seems like a normal behavior for people to do, but this is more of the norm than the exception.

I always smile and sometimes give a thumbs up. I mean, what else am I supposed to do? Hug them? Give a high-five? Give them a participation ribbon? How do I respond to this behavior? I have never really figured out the best response, but I'll say something like *you're almost there!* Maybe we share a laugh together and we go on about our lives. So strange. Welcome to my world.

I have literally never seen someone and thought, let me compare myself to them by getting on my knees. Doing this would feel awkward. For whatever reason when people see me, they think walking up to my shoulder and showing me where their head comes up to on my body is normal. Do I look like a measuring wall?! But I'm here for life, whatever that looks like, and I've stopped fighting it. In fact, I embrace it and believe it's comical.

There's something about us humans that makes us want to compare. Can you fault us? We start this world being compared. When you mom and dad sent out the baby announcement, they put how long you were and how much you weighed. Then, we think, *that's a good-sized baby*, or *that's a big baby*, or *how tiny*! We come into this world being measured so it's no wonder that we innately compare ourselves to throughout our lives.

Comparing is a cultural norm, we do this constantly in our daily lives.

- What store has lower prices?
- What company offers better benefits?
- Who's the breadwinner in the family?
- What auto repair can get the job done quicker?
- What hotel room has the better view?
- What vehicle has more trunk space?
- Which product has the best review?
- Which pair of shoes feels better?
- Where's the cheapest gas?
- Whose truck is taller? (ok- maybe that's just me because I want the tallest!)

We use these datapoints to help drive decisions and actions. What's the best move, the best purchase, the best area to focus on? If we choose the wrong thing, then we learn, we grow, we make different decisions. Life is nothing but data, and in order to make decisions we use analytics (comparisons) to determine the best path forward.

Makes sense why it's easy to want to compare ourselves to one another, it's what we know!

I remember getting into an elevator when I was in China. I'm not a big fan of getting in elevators with other people. I don't mind being tall, but elevators are so small. It feels unnatural to all be standing around silent, in a tiny space, with strangers breathing in my face. It's just weird. I get into this exceptionally tiny elevator and there's a family that's taking all the space around the perimeter. As I enter, I take a spot in the middle. Ugh. I feel like the goose in that game *Duck, Duck, Goose.* Not where I want to be standing. So, I'm there, and all of a sudden, I get a grab on my left cheek. Yes, someone has a handful of my butt cheek in their hand (I couldn't make this up if I wanted to). I cock my head, look over my left shoulder, and no joke, there's an 80-year-old woman laughing. We don't speak the same language, so she starts gesturing. She shows me where her head is in comparison to my body. Meanwhile, she's laughing, clearly amused by herself. So heck, I start laughing too. What on earth am I supposed to do other than laugh at this insane encounter.

I can respect this woman for being shorter, and she can respect me for being taller. I'm no better because I'm taller, and she's no better because she's shorter. Yes, we are different sizes, but that is fact. We are allowed to look at data, but keep facts as facts. My self-worth and value aren't determined by anyone else other than myself. You can compare facts, but they should not impact who you are, your value, your worth, how you see yourself. The only person that can set your value is you, and you're the only one you should be comparing yourself to.

You wouldn't look at a woman and a child and put them in them against each other in a marathon. The child can barely run. Their legs are tiny. They've not had time to train. There are so many reasons that come to mind that makes this scenario is foolish to consider. It should be obvious why these two shouldn't be compared to one another. And yet, we do this in our lives constantly.

- Who is more accomplished?
- Who makes more money?
- Who is more successful?
- Who has more followers?
- Who is higher up in the company?
- Who is more popular?

We are constantly mapping ourselves up to people in our industry, completely forgetting the iceberg effect.

When you're in the water and you look across the ocean, you only see the top. In the colder waters you might come across a piece of ice, an iceberg, that sticks out the top of the water. Any captain of a ship knows there's much more than meets the eye when you see ice sticking out of the water. You can only see 10% of the mass of ice, the other 90% is underwater and not visible above the surface. You want to avoid this mass if you're in a boat, it could be detrimental if you don't. This is like our lives; we only see people at a certain point in time (and often we notice once they've reached success). We see people when they're famous, or a CEO, or a business owner. What we don't see is all the hard work it took to get there, all the lessons along the way, all the heartache the person endured throughout their life to get to that point.

It's easy to look at someone, or that tip of the iceberg, and want what they have or compare yourself to where they are. But the truth is, we all have our own journey, our own stories, and our own path in life. Not one of us on this earth is going to have the same variables and journey. Just like that woman and child in the marathon, it doesn't make sense to compare. No two journeys are going to be the same, so why would you compare the end result?

I had a friend that got laid off once and she was bummed over the situation. It wasn't shortly thereafter that her mom got sick and she went to go take care of her. Over the next year, she began to understand and embrace the idea that her life was designed to help her mother while she was ill. They laughed, they traveled, they loved, they cried, and eventually her mother passed away. When I saw my friend again, there was a renewed glow to her. She was so grateful for the time she had with her mother and she knew that the universe had allowed her to spend this time with her mom.

After that year, my friend decided to take a different career path and coach professionals dealing with parents who are ill. It didn't make the same amount of money that she was making while in corporate, at first, but she was happy, she was fulfilled. Eventually, she began to be referred, her business grew, and she became a success story people talked about.

These were her variables that led her to having a successful business. There were lots of factors involved. It was the loss of her job, loss of her mother, it was an epiphany she had along the way to change careers. How do you compare to this? You don't. You shouldn't. This was her unique journey.

I have another friend who had a very successful career in finance. After a series of unfortunate events and bad decisions, he found himself in prison for three years. He lost everything. He was a family man who attended church, had a beautiful wife, a gorgeous daughter, a successful career, and yet he landed himself in prison. Fast forward to today, he is a well-known, contributing member to society. He plans massive events where he brings joy to people and families all over the Dallas area. Looking at him today, you would think he's well networked, successful, and loved; and he is! But his path to get there was a winding one with a lot of dark moments. You can't replicate the steps he took. This is his story, his journey, his path. Prison may have been the best thing that ever happened to him, but maybe not something any of us would volunteer for.

My sister, on the other hand, has had a pretty linear life. She went to college, married her college sweetheart, had a child, and worked her tail-off in a company for more than 10-years and became a Vice President. Her company was bought out, her department has gone through multiple rounds of lay-offs, and yet she retained her job throughout the consistent turnover.

Likely, it's because of her hard work, loyalty, leadership, personality, the value she adds, and her knowledge of the business that her company kept her. Pretty straight forward.

My story, on the other hand, is far from linear! I have a degree in Criminal Justice. I have an MBA. I worked as a leader in Information Technology for 15 years. I worked in Afghanistan for a year with a Top-Secret Clearance. I've been laid off a couple of times. I've gone through a divorce. Battled addictions. I've changed careers. I've lost money on real estate investments. I've had friends commit suicide. I've loved. I've lost. And despite it all, here I am. Today, I'm an author of multiple best-selling books, a motivational speaker, a certified coach, podcast host, I write for a magazine, I've been interviewed on all the major TV channels, I've interviewed some amazing public figures, my work has been published, I've been in numerous magazines, been to 49 countries...do I need to continue? How do you follow my path? And, to be entirely honest, there are people I could look at and compare myself to and it would look like I've done nothing.

But why?

Why do we compare ourselves to others when it's nothing more than a spider's web we get caught in? It's a trap. We need to remember that we all have our own unique story, so it's never going to be an apples-to-apples comparison. You will either feel you aren't enough, or you'll falsely inflate your ego against someone that doesn't appear to be as accomplished.

I was running a 5k with Irving Marathon in Irving, Texas and I started out alongside a friend of mine. At some point I decided I wanted to run a little faster, so I told him I was going to run ahead. I put my music on and focused on my steps and my breathing. I love running and there's something invigorating about pushing myself. Very often, I coach myself when I work out. *Atta girl! You can do this!* I'm usually saying something to encourage myself.

As I was running, I started to notice people passing me. I got caught in the spiders web. I started to compare myself to others. I saw how fast they were running and it put me into a state of suffering. I didn't feel good about my progress. What I didn't consider was the fact that many of these were probably trained runners, and I am not. I run, but I am more of a jogger, not a runner. I have no idea what is under their iceberg and what has gotten them to this point today. Is it even fair for me to think I should be comparing myself to people that might do this religiously and I only do it from time-to-time?

I also noticed something else that was happening as I started to focus on these other runners. I stopped coaching myself. As humans, we only have so much capacity as to where we put our attention. We don't have 5 verbal conversations at the same time, our brains don't work that way. We can have one at a time, maybe two, but we can't have our time and attention spread out in multiple avenues effectively. When I began to focus on the faster runners, I was not only feeling bad about myself, but I wasn't going as quickly as I could because I wasn't coaching myself. I lost my zone of focus because I was comparing myself to the other runners.

Fortunately, I caught myself. Even though I know not to compare, I got caught in the trap. When I realized what I was doing I immediately changed my thoughts. There was a funny thing that happened in that race. Turns out that for my age and sex I actually placed first! Go me! You are the only person you should compare yourself to.

- Are you better than you were yesterday?
- Are you making progress in your own life?
- Are you learning and growing?
- Are you evolving with life or are you stagnant?

Comparing yourself to someone else is like comparing apples to oranges. Not the same circumstances, variables, it's not fair to yourself, and it will kill or falsely elevate your confidence.

Celebrate your wins along the way, even if they seem small. This will help you to build your confidence. When you've accomplished a milestone or have that successful feeling—celebrate. Feeling successful doesn't have to be something extraordinary. Celebrate when you recognize limiting beliefs, when you acknowledge what you control versus don't control, or just when you have a good day. When you feel accomplished then you'll want that feeling again. You'll start to have faith and belief within yourself that you can do things. That you're capable of winning.

No matter how big or small, make sure you stand in your wins when they happen. If you glaze over them then you're robbing yourself of not only celebrating you, but also a chance to strengthen yourself and build confidence.

Your world is about you. They're the steps *you* take. The lessons *you* learn. The growth *you* experience. Your journey is irrespective of anyone else's. You grow when you're focused on you. You get caught in a spiders web when you're focused on others. Give yourself the attention you deserve and be the best Solitaire player you can be.

What makes you exceedingly valuable is there is only one of you! No one can be you. A Ferrari is more valuable than a Honda because there are less of them. Imagine if there was only one Ferrari, what do you think it would be worth? A lot. There is only one of you, that makes you invaluable.

Be who you were meant to be. Your story is uniquely designed for you. You have a journey that no one else can emulate. You weren't brought on this earth to copy someone else's journey, *you* are what makes you special. Stand in who you are. Don't compare.

Confidence is being secure in who you are, where you are, where you're headed, and accepting your journey. Stay in your lane and focus your eyes on the path you're trailblazing! In rowing, they have an expression, *keep your eyes in the boat*. Do not be distracted by what other are or are not doing.

You are the only one that is responsible for your happiness. Only you are responsible for your success. Only you are responsible for your confidence. And when you compare, you're sabotaging yourself, you may even find yourself going backwards.

As Thorin Klosowski says, "Don't compare your beginning with someone else's middle." Instead, compare yourself to yesterday. Strive for progress over perfection. You will build trust in your skills, your ability, your purpose when you stay in your lane and focus on what *you* set out to do. Build that confidence within yourself one celebratory brick at a time.

"A flower does not think of competing to the flower next to it. It just blooms."

— Zen Shin

Chapter 10: Practice, Practice, Practice!

Practice may or may not make perfect, but it's definitely going to get you more confident. It almost sounds cliché, but the only way to improve is to start. Ever seen a child take its first step? It is not the most graceful walk. In fact, after the child figures out how to stand and move with one foot in front of the other, it looks more like a waddle than a walk. But this is *huge* news! We tell our friends and family, announce it on social media, we get so proud of this child that took its first step! Major development! No one expects the child to have sturdy legs and begin running like a gazelle when it first stands up, it takes practice.

Why is it harder for us to apply that logic to our own lives? Maybe it's because we care what other people think. Maybe it's because we are so afraid of being judged, being rejected, or failing that we hold ourselves back.

Then, there's that imposter that will pop out and say *hello* from time-to-time and it tells you that you need to be perfect. That's a lot of pressure. I'm not even convinced perfect exits. You wouldn't put this pressure on a child, and you should have the same expectations for yourself.

If you saw a child fall down, would you tell it to give up? NO! You'd say everything was OK and to try it again. It's easier to give advice than to hold ourselves to it sometimes, but we are no different than children. We're just older and saggier. However you look, the same rules apply; it's going to be OK, you can do this, practice makes perfect.

Remember your brain learns through repetition. Once a path in your brain is created then it knows how to react or respond. There's less ambiguity, uncertainty, questioning, there's a definitive path that becomes the route you take. It's like ants going in and out of their ant hill, all walking one in front of the other like little robots. You don't see them deviating from the path; they're on a mission.

A few months after I started my last job in corporate, I moved to a new area of town. I didn't know this area whatsoever. It was a little southwest of Dallas, in an area called Oak Cliff (which gave me a lot of street cred for living there since it was a little rough around the edges). I bought a cute, old home that was built in 1917, and I was excited to be a homeowner in Dallas.

Since I was unfamiliar with this part of town, I took a different route to work for three weeks until I figured out the best commute. I relied on my GPS to get everywhere. I probably should have done a test run of my morning commute before I bought the place, but lesson learned. There were so many traffic lights and school zones that my commute took much longer than anticipated. I was determined to find the fastest route so I could avoid the daily bustle.

On one of the days I was trying a different route, I about jumped out of my skin as I navigated out of my area. Apparently, GPS wanted to take me on a street that changes traffic laws during certain hours of the day (I guess GPS didn't get the memo). As soon as I started to drive down this residential street, a woman in a very large, white Expedition drove head on toward me and blocked me from going forward. My first thought was from my terrorism training before I went to Afghanistan. I was ready to take my massive, diesel Ford F-250 with 35" tires and a lift and get her off the road (just as I was trained). But I kept my cool as she rolled her window down and started screaming at me.

"This is a one-way street!!! There are children!!!"

Oh. My. Goodness.

Momma Hen was in full force that morning protecting her chickadees!

Thank you, GPS! Next time, maybe get some updated information on when streets change to a one-way for a few hours! I hadn't noticed the sign either. There was so much happening on the street with kids and cars that I didn't see the sign with the hours listed.

I wanted to get the heck out of there as quickly as possible, but I couldn't just snap and disappear like this woman wanted me to- I'm not a genie, Karen!

My heart was racing. It's no wonder that we don't make the best decisions when we are in a state of suffering. My brain was in fight or flight mode and I had to force it to think rationally (which, I was trying to do, but Karen lost her mind and was totally aggressive). I'm lucky I got out of there without hurting myself or someone else. This woman had my nerves in a wad, and she was not making it easy for me to think. I made it out safely, but it honestly spun me up for a loop.

It took me hours to shake off the feelings of the morning and I wasn't thinking clearly until I calmed down. I kept getting triggered by this woman who beelined for me head on and cut me off while yelling at me.

I also programmed my brain that day. I learned one way NOT to go to work. As I was on my quest to find the best commute, this one was definitely off the table.

After three weeks, I found the best route and that became my daily commute. After a few more weeks, I no longer used my GPS and my brain went on autopilot on my drive into work.

Practice makes perfect (or at least gets you driving without your GPS). It takes time to find the optimal path, but you aren't going to know until you start.

You are going to run into situations, like mine with Karen, where you learn what not to do. Yes, they can be uncomfortable. Yes, they can be awkward to go through. Yes, they can even feel a little embarrassing. It's in those situations that you learn what not to do and you file that information away as data. Data, that's all your brain is processing. Don't go down a one-way street. Check. Got it. It's also an opportunity to assess your beliefs. Remember, we talked about our beliefs being the root of our experience, so if you are in a state of suffering then look at the beliefs supporting those feelings.

I believed this woman was aggressive, she triggered me to believe she could be a threat. My initial response was to get her out of my way, but I choose to have control over my thoughts. I chose to change the response (the habit) because I could see the unintelligent thinking in my belief system. I chose to believe that instead of a threat, she was a concerned mother that would do anything to protect her children. She was responding in the way she believed was the solution.

It takes 21-days to change a habit, so keep doing what you're doing and eventually it will become second nature. You will start to have more confidence in your skills and your ability when you train your brain what to do. You won't think about using your GPS, how to walk, how to sell, how to be a good friend, how to walk up and talk to someone—it will come naturally!

With enough practice, your brain will become comfortable with the path it created. Keep in mind that the first time you do something it may feel wobbly or imperfect, but this will improve. This is the discomfort we talked about. You have to go through growth to get to the goal. Know that this is a normal part of the process and embrace the feeling. Keep practicing so you develop a habit and it becomes natural for you.

What's something you're good today? Think about a first time you gave it a try. Were you as confident and polished as you are today? You may have been reserved, timid, uncertain, scared, you may have had all sorts of feelings and emotions. Then, you practiced and it got easier. You weren't as nervous, you didn't question your abilities, you started to perform with ease. Think back on this time and see how far you came with practice. You did it once, you can certainly do it again! Remind yourself of this as you venture into something new-- you're more than capable!

Focus on the positives. Focus on what it going well. Tell yourself that this could happen and that will elevate the faith you have in what you're doing. Confidence is a positive emotion; don't polarize it with negativity. We know that where your thoughts go, your energy flows, so choose your thoughts wisely. Imagine what it will look like when you've become proficient. Manifest this person. See this person in flow with confidence and it will become you with practice.

~~~

Practicing is going to help you not only feel more confident but will help you reach a level of mastery, the two go hand-in-hand.

Tony Schwartz, CEO of The Energy Project, says, "Confidence equals security equals positive emotion equals better performance." In other words, when we have confidence then we are more secure in what we do. When we feel secure then we have more positive emotions. Positive emotions help us to perform better. You are an ecosystem and what you put into yourself matters. Time, messaging, practice, people you surround yourself by, food- it all matters and will impact your output and your overall health.

I'd suggest eliciting feedback from people you trust and respect. Let go of the idea of perfection, leave your ego at the door, and ask people you trust how you can improve. Those that truly love and care for you, those that have an interest in your success and wellbeing can help you improve your game.

I was asked to attend a seminar from a woman that had put together a course on *Mining Your Brilliance*. There was a group of us that agreed to participate in this full day course. As she went through her curriculum, there were times she pointed out that something was out of order. She also realized that what she had put together was going to take longer than the eight hours she had originally anticipated. At the end of the day, she elicited feedback from each of the participants.

Genius. This woman's process was spot on! First, she didn't have an ego about her course being perfect. She even mentioned in the beginning that she believed it was better to practice and improve than to wait until it was perfect to roll out. She understood the importance of practice and surrounding herself with a group of trusted individuals. She knew this group would be able to provide her with honest and trustworthy feedback. She didn't have to take our feedback, but she trusted us enough to at least consider our input.

Now, she's practiced, she has positive feedback, she's able to make modifications to her curriculum, and it's closer to being ready to roll out to the public.

Practice. Practice. Practice! And getting feedback is so valuable! You don't need to guess what people want, like, need—simply ask a sample of people you trust!

Remember, everyone is entitled to their opinion and has their own set of beliefs. You don't have to take the suggestions, they're ultimately your call.

Practice doesn't have to be in front of people, you can do it in the comfort of your own home or by yourself. Play the guitar in your garage and pretend you're up on stage. Speakers can practice in front of the mirror or talking to a collective of chairs in their house. Practice asking someone on a date by talking to your animal.

You can even practice just using your imagination! Dr. David Hamilton conducted a study of piano players practicing the piano. He did a brain scan when the players had their fingers on the keyboard and when they imagined their hands on the keyboard. The brain had the same response. Therefore, he concludeed that the brain cannot distinguish the difference between real and imaginary.

~~~

As Tony Schwartz so eloquently stated, confidence gives security, positive emotions, and better performance. Practicing is one of the most basic ways to become confident. Don't expect perfection from the start. *Practice makes perfect,* not, *perfect comes on your first try*.

Assess your belief system as you get into action. When you experience suffering (internal dissonance), get to the core of your thoughts and what are the beliefs behind them? If they don't serve you—change them.

Remember, it takes 21-days to form a habit. Keep practicing so your brain knows the proper response to the commands you give.

Allow yourself room to grow and give yourself grace. Put that ego to the side. All good things come with time, so give yourself that permission to evolve.

Ask people their opinions and make improvements if you want to incorporate their suggestions.

Practice in the quiet of your own home. Practice using your imagination. Practice in front of trusted peers and watch your confidence clime as you go for primetime.

Mastery comes by starting; it doesn't come at the start. The more you practice, the more confident you'll become. There's no circumventing this step, you have to walk through the fire to get through the other side. It will get easier, just keep at it!

I end every podcast episode on *Level Up To 2.0* by saying, "The only way to level up....is to do the work!" Get out there and do the work! It will get easier. It will become second nature! Practice. Practice. Practice!

"Inaction breeds doubt and fear. Action breeds confidence and courage. If you want to conquer fear, do not sit home and think about it. Go out and get busy."

-Dale Carnegie

Chapter 11: Meeting Yourself Where You're At

High achievers have high expectations of themselves. They also have high output. I'm a high achiever, so I know. This is where, when I see the next peak of the mountain, I get intrigued, and I aim for it. Then, I see the next one and go for it. If I gut punched, no problem, I just keep going. When I am laser focused on something, nothing can stop me.

Is this you?

Do you get in a vortex of cranking out accomplishments? Do you find yourself constantly seeking that next big thing to put a check mark next to that you've completed?

When I stepped out of my corporate career, I was immediately humbled. I had a lot to learn.

I've always had a lot to learn, all of us do. We don't come walking out the womb with all the answers, we learn it as we go. I felt confident in my corporate career, but as I became an entrepreneur, I realized there was a lot to learn. I had to learn all the functions in every department, many of which I had no idea how to do. Stepping into this new role was a ride I didn't expect and I had to learn to meet myself where I was at.

Confidence can be shaken when you try new things. Even if you're a high performer, it doesn't always mean you have solid footing when you try something new. That imposter syndrome may surface. You might get uncomfortable. You might want to go back to your lane of expertise so you feel like a high achiever again.

I began my dream business as a side-hustle while I was still in corporate. After I was laid off at the beginning of COVID, my world of success and accomplishments appeared to take a sharp turn. I now had a baby business and more expenses than real income! Gone were the days of a predictable paycheck- it was time to bring my vision to life!

No one could have prepared me for what I jumped into as I began to build my business. I definitely did not get a job description like I did when I got hired in corporate. My corporate position was spelled out for me, including my annual goals and overall responsibilities. I would be assessed twice a year by my boss to see if I was on target. At the end of the year, I would get a final review of my performance and deliverables. Although there was a lot to learn in corporate and it was often chaotic, it was more predictable and laid out. I was in my lane of expertise.

Being an entrepreneur is a bit like jumping off a cliff and building your parachute on the way down. You might not have any idea what you're doing, but you better figure something out. No job description. No single job function. Just pieces of a parachute to put together as you jump off that cliff into a world unknown.

With the exception of the CEO (and maybe an internal auditor), when you start a traditional corporate job you are assigned to a department. You don't get assigned to all the departments, just the one. Each department plays a critical role in the overall operation. When you become an entrepreneur (and let's start with being a solopreneur, like I was), you get to learn every single department. You're now a marketer, a website designer, a business development manager, an IT specialist, a security manager, the operations manager, legal, the CFO, you're everything. I know a lot about a lot of things, but there were a TON of things I knew nothing about.

I had no idea how to build a website, create funnels, develop courses, copywrite, build a brand, social media, grow a following, and public relations. I never had to do any of these in my past life. And yes, you can outsource anything, but when you're just getting started it doesn't make sense to outsource everything. One of my first unfamiliar tasks; build a website.

Learning to build a website was no joke. I worked in Information Technology for 15-years and yet my technical skills were at about a 1 or 2 on the scale of 1-10 (1 being the lowest). Yes, I led IT teams, but I knew who did what and who would get things done, I wasn't the doer.

As a new entrepreneur, however, I was the doer.

In a sense, I felt like I went back in time and was 20 again. I was that young girl, sitting in the bar in Germany, not knowing anything about life, but laughing with the German that was hugging me on a ladder. I was just figuring out my direction in life and my confidence. Now, I was in my mid-thirties and I was learning a new world again.

When you're a high achiever, you want forward momentum. It's what you're familiar with. You feel accomplished with a high level of output. Pivoting into a new lane is going to come with a learning curve, and the initial output will look different.

The challenge was, I had tasted one definition of success. I had lived one definition of victory. I had accomplished a lot. And now, well, I was figuring out how I could make something out of nothing and build a website with no skills and no budget. I was building a business with no guidance. I was researching hashtags and becoming obsessed with number of likes and how many followers I had. I was taking courses on how to use Instagram (I should have learned from a 5-year-old instead of the $300 course I bought from some chick online). No paycheck and I'm obsessed with likes on Instagram. What on earth am I doing with my life?!

There was a lot of investing in myself I needed to do as well. Coaching programs became my biggest expense, I invested in me all along the way. This helped because I could not only get support, but I could also be with others on a similar path. I definitely wasn't alone on this entrepreneurial rollercoaster and wasn't the only one starting out amidst a pandemic!

I realized a very important lesson as soon as I was immersed in my dream full-time. I had to learn to meet myself where I was at. I needed to be patient and kind with myself. I may not have been in the board room talking about million-dollar budgets and initiatives, but I was still doing big things. What's the definition of *big things,* anyhow? You get to decide, quite frankly.

Just as we talked about comparing yourself to others kills your confidence, same is true when you compare yourself to other points along your life's timeline. It's true, the only person you want to compare yourself to is yourself, but your life is also dynamic. The variables of yesterday are going to be different than tomorrow, so life isn't always going to take a steady incline. What does *incline* even mean?

I may manage a team of individuals at age 40, but I may not want to manage anyone when I turn sixty. Does that mean it's a step back? Does that mean I'm less successful? No, it means I'm at a different point in my life and I want different things. I may decide that managing people is too much work and drama and I'd rather not deal with all that. It's in no way an indication on my success, but rather a change in where I'm at in my life. In fact, I may define success at 60 as working as little as possible. Be in flow with your life and do what works for you at each stage.

Life is ever evolving and you need to be ready to bob and weave as life moves. Learn to be in the flow of life. Every boxer knows that if you stand still, you're bound to get punched. Let go of what you can't control and focus on what you can control. When the uncontrollable happens, you may need to shift. This is not a reflection of being unsuccessful, but rather it's wise if you can learn to be in the flow rather than resisting. Meet yourself here. You're doing the best you can and always keep building toward that purpose.

What worked for you yesterday may not work for you tomorrow, and that doesn't mean you've gone backwards, you're just at a different place. You get to define your success. You get to define your happiness. You get to choose your beliefs. Life is fluid. Meet yourself and adapt your definitions and expectations along your life's journey. Compare yourself to where you were yesterday to whatever goal you're currently set out to achieve.

~~~

Confidence is trusting in yourself. It's believing in what you're doing, it's knowing that everything is going to be OK. If I had held myself to the same level of output as I had when I was in corporate on day one of my entrepreneurial journey, not only would it have been unfair, but it would have also diminished my confidence. I would have been asking:

- Am I good enough?
- Should I be on this path?
- Am I doing it right?
- What will people think of me?
- Am I a failure?
- Can I pull this off?

So, I had to pivot my baseline of expectations and meet myself right where I was standing. I was giving 110% to what I was doing, that's what I needed to be focused on. Was I making progress and speaking into my purpose? Was I being true and authentic to myself? Was I happy? Was I making the impact I wanted to make? These were the more powerful questions I needed to be asking myself.

It's easy to get focused on the end state goal, but it's truly the journey we learn from, grow from, and find joy. What happens when you get focused on the end state goal and not the journey? When you achieve the goal then you set another, and another, and another. If you are only focused on celebrating the *big wins* then you're going to miss the moments that are happening along the way. As Dr. Seuss said it best, "sometimes you will never know the value of a moment, until it becomes a memory." If we're only focused on the end state goal, then what teaching moments have you missed? What growth did you overlook? What joy did you miss?

Enjoy the journey. Celebrate your wins. Meet yourself where you're at. This isn't a competition; life is to be enjoyed.

Don't be afraid to pivot in life or try something new. When you pivot, modify your expectations and definitions to serve where you're at.

I went to a friend's house one day and her dad was there. He asked what I had been up to. He knew I left corporate and was on my own journey. I was excited to announce that I had just rolled out my first online mindset course!

The first thing that came out of his mouth was, "so how much money have you made?" That was one of those *excuse me* moments. I realized that we had two very different perceptions of the situation. His definition of success clearly came in the form of money. When I looked at the situation, this signified how far I had come from my starting point within my own personal journey, not just when I left corporate. I was so proud of myself because I knew how much work I had done. I could see how much I had grown as a human and the dedication I had to myself and my dreams. I knew the 27 different job functions I played in order to get to that point. I didn't care if I hadn't made money yet, I was floored at my success!

I learned an important lesson that day. Not only do you need to meet yourself where you're at, but not everyone is going to see your vision. Not everyone can see your potential. Not everyone is going to support you. The only person that can truly support you is you.

My inner confidence had to be stronger than this force of perceivable judgement. I needed to have that trust, that belief, that security within myself to stand up for my dream and what I was doing.

You are no better and no less than anyone else. Everyone is on their own journey and we're at different points with different variables. People may project their opinions on you. You may have an idea of where you need to be. The truth is, you are right where you are supposed to be, even if you hit a reset button in your life (which we'll talk about later).

Being a part of the journey is going to allow you to learn, grow, and enjoy those small moments. Let's eradicate this idea of where you should be and focus on doing the best right where you're at. Doesn't matter the size or the magnitude, you are right where you need to be. Give life your all and aim to be a little better tomorrow (if it's the same path you took today).

At the end of the day, you have to believe in you. No one can propel you through this life. No one can make that decision to get you out of bed, to pull your head back into the game, to go do something new. You are the only one responsible for your happiness, your success, your life.

I choose to meet myself where I am every moment of every day. I don't need to compare myself to anyone else or take on anyone else's definition of success. If I gave it my all and I made a small stride one day, I focus on doing it better and faster the next.

Meeting yourself where you're at helps you to not just boost your confidence, but to also have more enjoyment in life. You're tapped into the moment versus living in the future. You're able to appreciate and be grateful. You're learning in the present and able to make incremental steps forward. There's no lack, no shame, but rather an appreciation for every step of the way. You're focused on building a sturdy path; one foot in front of the other.

"Everyone wants to live on top of the mountain, but all the happiness and growth occurs while you're climbing it."

-Andy Rooney

Chapter 12: Failure is a Choice

Failure is one of my favorite topics to talk about, which sounds a little cuckoo-for-cocoa-puffs, but I love talking to someone about their failures. I enjoy asking someone to think about a time they failed. There's an energy shift that happens. No one wants to think about a time that they failed! It's embarrassing. It's sad. It's angry. It's resentful. It doesn't feel good. Failure is a lack of success, and who doesn't want to succeed?

Failure makes us feel like we did something wrong. So why is this one of my favorite topics? Because when you realize it's a belief that you own then you can make a different choice. You know by now that you own your beliefs and your beliefs create your experience in life. If you want a different experience then you need to change your belief. That's the power of choice. That's the power of the mind. If something doesn't serve you, then make a different choice.

Failure is just a word, all words are just words. It's the association and meaning we give to words that gives them definition.

Let's look at the word *scrubber.* What comes to mind?

For me, I think about scrubbing toilets or scrubbing dishes. I think of the apparatus one would use to do the act of scrubbing. Or you are a person that scrubs and therefore you are a scrubber. Pretty benign word, not really significant. If I heard my dad telling my mom that she was the scrubber that night, I would assume she was washing the dishes.

In the British language, however, *scrubber* is a promiscuous woman. It might be someone that is scrubbing dishes, but it is also someone that is promiscuous, like the word *whore*. It would be an entirely different conversation if this was the meaning of the word that my father was using versus doing the dishes (which he would never do, just to clarify).

How about the word *pup*? I think of a dog, maybe even a little dog, more like a puppy. I think of a soft, excited, tiny puppy that is less than a year old and still has that cute look. I might even go as far to think about a young kid, but probably not the first association I would make with this word. In Ireland, *pup* is like a *brat* or a *prick*. It's a derogatory word someone would use to tear someone down.

Butter. Seems pretty straight forward. I think of the sticks or the tubs of churned cream that they sell in the stores and you put it on toast or to cook with. Butter is delicious, especially when my scallops are seared in them with a splash of salt. I love butter! In New Zealand, however, if you're called *butter*, then you have a hot body but your face is ugly. Butter is not a kind word in New Zealand so be careful if you tell someone they are *smooth like butter*.

My point is, words are words and we create the meaning and association. Meaning matters. If you get called a *pup, butter scrubber*, it might not mean that you are a puppy that's scrubbing butter. Rather, you've just been called a *prick of a woman that has a good body and an ugly face that's also a whore*. Meaning matters.

If we have the ability to change the meaning of words, then we should, shouldn't we? Failure is not something that makes you feel good, so change it.

I'd argue that failure is one of three things:

1. It's a lesson(s) learned
2. It's a course correction
3. Combination of lesson(s) and course correction

Whatever the outcome, your goal is to grow.

If you believe the definition of failure to be negative, then you'll look at the situation as having been defeated. Confidence deflates when you feel defeated. We talked about limiting beliefs, and if you believe failure is negative, then you may believe the following to be true if you put yourself out there and don't succeed:

- People will look down on me.
- My family will be disappointed.
- They'll laugh at me.
- They'll be mad at me.
- They won't be able to trust me again.
- My career will be ruined.
- I won't ever be happy again.
- I won't be worthy of being loved.
- I'll never get this opportunity again.

There are a million beliefs that could go through your mind before or after a situation. These are the thoughts that will hold you back from experience life, maybe even trying! And, how could they not? If you believed everyone would hate you if you didn't succeed- that's heavy! Knowing you're going to be OK and believing in yourself and your mission feels a whole heck of a lot better!

Do these beliefs serve you?

They don't.

Let's say you had the confidence to put yourself out there to the world. You tried and it didn't turn out the way you wanted it to. Now what?

Some questions you should be asking yourself are:

- What did I learn?
- What went well?
- What didn't go well?
- What could go better next time?
- Was there someone I should have talked to beforehand?
- Did I have the right people engaged?
- Did I ask the right questions up front?
- Is this the path I'm supposed to be on?

It's just data you're assessing. There's nothing you can do about the past. The only time you can truly control is the here and now. You can forge the path for tomorrow, but today is the only time frame you can actually control. It's a choice to look at a situation and grow from what you learned. This is the growth mindset. When you know better-- do better.

Failure doesn't exist.

Have you ever gone on WebMD to try to self-diagnose yourself? You may have the common cold, but by the time you're done researching you believe you're dying. Your common cold becomes more and more severe as you start to research (even if your symptoms haven't changed). Our minds are like gravity and negativity is a weight. Negativity will hold you down and keep you on that trajectory until you hit bottom. Confidence is a positive emotion that sets you free and is limitless. You can't have weights and fly (or maybe you can, but you won't fly as high).

Negativity is a downward spiral. The first step to overcome it is to catch it when it shows up. Negativity is telling you something bigger is happening under the surface. It could be unresolved pain, anger, frustration that has never been dealt with. When negativity arises, notice it. Acknowledge where your brain is leading you and take control. Does this serve me (I sound like a broken record)? If not, look at your beliefs.

Think about an actual situation that didn't work out. Think about it for a minute until something comes to mind. Feel what's happening in your body. Pay attention to your emotions. Did you get a divorce? Did your kid do something horrendous? Did you buy a house, but you got in way over your head? Did you have to file for bankruptcy? Did you forget the words to your presentation?

How are you feeling right now?

If you're feeling negative, park those feelings.

What did you learn from that experience? How did you grow? Did you find strength you didn't know you had? What do you now have or now know because you went through the situation?

Now, tell yourself you didn't fail. Failure doesn't exist. Failure is a word and you get to choose the meaning. The meaning of failure is to teach you, to grow you, to guide you to where you're supposed to be. Ask yourself:

- What could I have done differently?
- What went well?
- Are there areas within myself that I can improve upon?
- Is there anyone I could have consulted with?
- Were there other options?
- Would I do it again with a set of different knowledge?
- What knowledge would I need in order to do it again?
- What questions or steps could I have taken before that would have possibly yielded a different outcome?

It feels more like data, doesn't it? It's data that you're getting from the situation that you're analyzing. It's not a reflection on you, but rather it's data to build on. Look at the facts, not the beliefs. If the beliefs are negative, change them.

How does the situation feel now?

Sure, it might still sting a bit. It doesn't feel good to go into bankruptcy, fold your business, forget the words in your presentation, get a divorce, go to jail, if your mind is focused on them being failures.

Let's say you got a divorce. I know, I've been there, doesn't feel all that good. You walked down the aisle with someone. You went in thinking it was going to last forever, we all do, but it didn't. When this happened to me I thought this was a massive black mark on my dating resume. I was never going to be able to check the *SINGLE* box again for my status, it was always going to be the status of *DIVORCE*. Gross. How could I be a divorced 30-year-old? What did that say about me? What would the guys think about me? Would they think that I wasn't datable because I was already divorced? To be honest, I felt like damaged goods.

Turns out, that was all just a mindset.

I love the song by Garth Brooks (this may be the third book I've written about this song), *Unanswered Prayers*. He talks about how he prayed and prayed to have this woman in his life. His prayers went unanswered. I'm sure he was down and out about it, he wanted her so badly he was praying to God to have her in his life. God, however, had a different plan. Instead of the woman he was praying for, God gave him another woman, and this woman was the love of his life. His *Unanswered Prayers* allowed him to meet the real woman of his dreams. He never would have met his soulmate had he married the first woman.

There is a design for your life, a greater plan, a master plan, and you can't see it. None of us can see the master plan. Sure, we can close our eyes and imagine what it will look like, but we don't actually know what is going to happen. We don't have a Magic 8-Ball that tells us the answers or a way to see the future. When we go into an endeavor, we believe it's going to work out. When we walk down the aisle, we believe the marriage will last. When we start a company, we believe it will be successful. When we buy a house, we believe it will be a good investment. We don't walk into these situations thinking they will tank, but sometimes they do.

I remember when I got laid off from my last corporate company. Getting laid off can be blindsiding. You may have an idea that it's coming, but you may have no idea. When I was laid off, my phone blew up with people telling me how much the company sucked and how sorry they felt for me. I think I was the only one that wasn't in a state of suffering or feeling sorry over the situation. This wasn't a failure and I wasn't a victim. This wasn't a loss; it was an opportunity! I was ready to take on the next phase of my life and I embraced the cards that were dealt. There's nothing I could do about the situation, so I might as well embrace it with open arms rather than put up a fight. It was time to pursue my dreams full-time, and that was the immediate decision I made. No suffering, no failure, I saw opportunity.

Failure doesn't feel good, it impacts your confidence. When things happen differently than you expect, embrace the opportunity. Find the silver lining. Look for the lesson. The world is working for you, not against you, if you choose to see it and respond to it that way.

Failure is a belief that you control. You give the meaning to words and you can change them if you want. Failure is one of my favorite topics because it's one that trips so many people up and yet it's easy to turn around. We can get paralyzed by this idea of failure and go hide in a cubby hole. Our ego gets hurt. Our confidence gets shattered. But it doesn't have to if we change the way we look at the situation.

If you believe that failure is negative then it can hold you back from being confident. Look for the lessons. Look for the course corrections. In either situation (or they could be both), grow, and always be growing. They say if you aren't growing, you're dying.

It's OK to be a pup, butter scrubber- if you give it the right meaning!

"Failures are finger posts on the road to achievement."

- C.S. Lewis

Chapter 13: Making Confident Decisions

They say there are a million ways to skin a cat. I don't know who came up with that bizarre saying, but considering I have a cat, I find that saying a little odd.

Neither here nor there, but it's saying there are lots of different decisions you can make to accomplish a goal. How many options do you have for dinner? How many career choices do you have?   How many ways are there to fold laundry? What do you want to do with your Friday night? Where do you want to take your next vacation? How do you want to wear your hair? What do you want to name your child? So many decisions!

How do you decide?

The decision-making process can be overwhelming. It used to be that the occupational choices were minimal for women, mainly teachers, nurses, or secretaries. Now, women can be anything they want to be- they can be a man if that's what they choose! Skies the limit!

With so many options, how do we stay confident in the decisions we make? How do we know if we're making the right decisions?

The fear of the unknown, the possibility of making the wrong decision, the potential to make a mistake keeps many people from taking action. They tell themselves it's safer to stay in a place they're familiar with than face any kind of failure, rejection, or mistake. Your brain is wired to keep you safe and it's uncomfortable when it goes into new territory.

Should you ask someone on a date?

Should you even approach the person to talk to?

Should you write that book?

Should you change jobs?

Should you travel by yourself?

Should you travel abroad?

Should you move?

If you do move, where should you go? Should you buy a house? Should you rent? Do you want a house with a pool? Do you need to live close to your job? Do you need to be near an airport? Do you want a two-story home? One-story home? Do you need a fence in the backyard? You may commit to the idea of moving, but there are so many decisions that come after that it has you retreating back right to where you started.

How do you make confident decisions when there are so many to choose from? Truth is, it can be so overwhelming that you shut down and do nothing. Have you been there? Does that serve you to do nothing? When you're 80, I want you to look back and have zero regrets. Inaction, overwhelm, and fear will not get you to your goals; confidence will.

We know confidence is a mindset. It's self-assurance, it's knowing everything is going to be OK, it's the trust and belief in yourself. When you make a decision, apply these same beliefs. Whatever you choose, it's going to be OK. Trust it's the right move. Believe that it was the right decision with the information you had.

Having confidence in your decisions doesn't mean everything will work out the way you think it will. It means you are able to make a decision, get into action, and stand behind this direction.

Think of a leader you have high admiration for. What qualities about their guidance, leadership, direction are appealing? It's the leader's role to share the vision with the team and lead them in a direction. A leader has the right to change direction, but a good leader is going to be very strategic and minimal when doing so. It creates confusion for the team when the vision isn't clear and the direction is fluid.

You are your own leader. You are the only one that is creating your path forward to fulfill your dreams, your goals, your destiny. First and foremost, inaction will get you nowhere. A good way to look back in life and wonder if you coulda, shoulda, woulda is to do absolutely nothing. You need to start with a decision.

Worried about everyone else?

It's natural to wonder what others are going to think, what they'll say, if they'll judge. We have to remember these are just opinions, and everyone is entitled to their own opinions and beliefs. It doesn't mean they have to align with yours. Opinions aren't facts. Don't hold yourself back because you're concerned about an opinion that someone formed based on their own belief system. You know you can't please everyone, so why hold yourself back?

Let's look at the decisions the new CEO of a company was faced with.

The CEO comes into work her first day and tells her staff that she needs to cut the headcount by 10%. It's not an easy conversation to have to let employees go and it can be hard on morale. The leadership team comes up with a plan and the next week they execute on the reduction.

At lunch, two employees start talking about the situation.

> **Employee 1:** "Good way to start out her time here, way to really get people to like you! Just fire the staff- that will make them want to work for you! She doesn't care about us. I'm sure she'll be happy getting her bonus!"

> **Employee 2:** "Well, that might be, but I heard the Board gave her an ultimatum. Someone in Finance told me that she didn't have a choice."

> **Employee 1:** "You honestly think she didn't have a choice?"

> **Employee 2:** "Who knows, maybe, but no one can be worse than the last yahoo that was here, he was an idiot!"

> **Employee 1:** "Yeah. He was literally the worst CEO ever!"

Lots of opinions from Employee #1.

1. Firing people will make the rest of the employees not like you.
2. The new CEO doesn't care about the employees.
3. Firing employees means you don't care about employees.
4. The CEO made the choice to have the reduction in force.

5. The last CEO was the worst CEO ever!

Employee #2 tried to introduce facts, at least what she understood to be true, that the Board gave the CEO an ultimatum.

It's easy as a bystander to look at a situation and draw an opinion. It's not easy being the CEO, the President, the Head of State, the parent, the one that makes the decisions. You just aren't going to please everyone.

The fact of the situation with the CEO was that when she signed on with the company, she told them that she would help the company save money. Her first approach would be to cut budget, not headcount. She would entertain a reduction in force only after she was embedded in the company for at least 90-days. Before she came on board, however, a consulting company had come in and completed a headcount assessment. Numbers were too high. Employees were sitting around doing nothing and there wasn't enough work to substantiate their employment. Their recommendation was a 15% headcount reduction.

The Board announced that upon her starting, the new CEO was going to need to make this reduction immediately. Although reluctant, she agreed to a 10% reduction. She also agreed to make up the financial impact of the remaining 5% by reducing the bonuses across the board by one percent. This way she was able to retain 5% of the staff until she could make her own assessment on productivity. Yes, she would have to deal with the whiplash of the 1% reduction in bonuses, but she felt better about reducing the bonus instead of more people. She might make a different judgement call after she was able to assess the company, but she felt good in the decisions she made.

The CEO knew she wasn't going to make everyone happy. In fact, it wasn't what she had originally intended to do in her first 90-days with the company. You aren't always going to be given variables that you want to work with, but rather what you have to work with. At the end of the day, she was going to need to make decisions. If the Board disapproved her suggestion, then she was either going to have to proceed forward or leave; she landed on the compromise that felt best and they agreed.

Although the CEO didn't want to layoff anyone right away, she stood behind the decisions she made. She trusted that the situation was going to work out and she believed in her abilities to manage situations through completion. Not her first rodeo as a leader, she could certainly get through a small reduction in force.

She made a decision and moved forward believing in her abilities as a leader.

Life isn't always going to hand you a situation where you have the option of making everyone happy.

- Kids might not like curfews the parents implement; other kids might understand they're for their own good.
- Most of the staff won't like layoffs; others might be glad they cut out people that we're contributing.
- Some citizens disagree with going to war; or they might think there's no other way to protect the country.
- Some people don't want tax dollars to be spent on NASA and exploring space; others might believe we are setting ourselves up for failure if we aren't on the bleeding edge of space exploration.
- Some people believe guns should be banned; others believe they're our right.

You aren't always going to win. There are too many opinions and beliefs of how things *should be.*

Back to the CEO and the reduction in force. There was no one answer that was going to fit for everyone, so she had to make a decision based on what she believed to be best. She may learn along the way that there are better ways of handling the situation, but she'll only know once she tries. When you know better-- do better. Or maybe that was absolutely the right thing to do in the first place. A leader, in any capacity, is to make decisions and stand behind them. If there is fall out, then clean it up. If it goes well, then repeat it again in the future when you need to.

Why can it be so hard to make decisions?

There are lots of reasons.

Many of us are people-pleasers and quite possibly you want to make everyone happy. Or you don't want to upset anyone and rocking the boat is too scary. Maybe it's that you want to be accepted by others, so you feel you need to adapt to what they want or what they like. Maybe making a decision is too much work. Maybe making a decision seems too scary.

What would you do if you found out you're allergic to seafood? You wouldn't repeat it, would you? With the new data you have of knowing you're allergic, you now should take that into consideration going forward. The next time you're at a party and there's seafood being served then you should avoid it altogether. Let's say, you accidentally eat something that has small traces of seafood and you didn't know. You get sick. Next time, you make sure to ask the host if there's anything you're allergic to in any of the food. Over time, you get really good about avoiding the foods that are going to make you sick, but it was a process to get wise about.

It's the same as anything you do. Do the best you can with the information you have and move forward.

I bought a piece of property in Dallas once and I was planning on building my dream home. I went and checked out the property, did my research on the price per square foot, I looked at the neighborhood and saw the property value increasing. I honestly thought I had done my research. I bought the property, tore down the old house, and quickly learned that I was in a mess.

When I tore the house down, the property got automatically rezoned commercial and I had to fight to get it rezoned back to residential with the county. This took four months of my time and a lot of money. Then, I found out that it was in the 100-year floodplain. This was going to have me jumping through even more hoops. Oh, did I mention I had already bought the plans to the house without ever knowing if I was going to be able to fit that house on that property? I made a lot of decisions that I learned from, but now I know.

I made the decisions, I learned from them, I grew from them, and I know better what to do next time. Even in imperfect situations, you can still have confidence. It goes back to the fundamental definition. You have the belief, trust, and security in knowing that you can navigate any situation, even if it doesn't turn out the way you think it will. I didn't anticipate this situation happening, but my world didn't fall apart because of the decision I made; I recovered.

I'm not advocating to be reckless in your decisions. Had I asked better questions, done more research, done different research, then the outcome very well could have been different. But I did the best I could with what I knew, and I didn't know I needed to ask better questions. Now I know. Do the best you can with what you know. When you know better—do better.

~~~

The trick is getting started. There are lots of reasons that could get in your way, but whose life are you building; yours or someone else's? Whose happiness are you responsible for? Who will have the regrets later in life if no action or forward movement is taken?

Go back to what it felt like for you have belief and trust in yourself. Imagine your life with confidence. Imagine how it felt. Visualize how you would show up. Yes, it can be overwhelming to make a decision, but if you don't, then nothing will change. Whatever your life looks like now is how it will stay. Those goals you want to reach and the person you want to be will stay in your head.

The world isn't going to fall apart because of a decision you made. You don't have the divine power to make the world stop. Think about your last crisis or *failed* project. You made it through, didn't you? The world didn't fall apart, and it's not going to this time either.

Tell yourself it could happen. I mean, if Meghan Markle can marry a prince then anything can happen! Instead of, telling yourself *it won't happen*, replace that with *it could happen*! This is faith. Believe it can!

Make sure you stay aligned with your personal values and beliefs. If you know who you are then you are better prepared for any situation. If someone starts gossiping to you and gossip doesn't align with your values, then walk away. You will be able to make a more confident decision if you know who you are. When you know yourself then you know how to navigate situations. You still may wonder what you want for dinner, but knowing your values and beliefs will help you to confidently stand when some major decisions and bigger situations come your way.

Be your own coach and ask yourself powerful questions (or find a mentor and/or coach). Ask yourself:

- What's the outcome if I do?
- What's the outcome if I don't?
- What's the risk?
- What's the reward?
- How will this make me feel?

It's not always about how quickly you can make a decision, but rather making the best decision with the information you have in an appropriate amount of time. Once you make a decision, move forward with confidence. If you need to change along the way, make a change, but do it minimally and strategically.

I think of that show, *Who Wants To Be A Millionaire*:

"Final answer?"

"Yes, final answer."

Make your decision and move forward.

As the world presents itself, move in flow. You can neither predict nor control what is going to happen tomorrow, so stand solid in where you're at today.

Don't seek external validation to keep you afloat, that's an unpredictable source of elevation. You control the trust and faith you have within yourself- don't rely on other's to fill your cup.

Confidence is internal. It's nice to get a compliment, to hear you've done well, to get positive feedback, but this should just be the bonus. Focus on your beliefs, your values, your goals, your dreams.

Confident decision making is sticking to a decision and moving forward. You open yourself to learning and growing along the way as you move forward with your decision. When it's the right time to change, you'll know.

No one said that making decisions was going to be easy; no one said that it had to be hard either. Both are beliefs and you choose which one you want to believe. What matters is the belief in yourself that no matter what you decide, you can get through everything.

Life is nothing more than a bunch of decisions stacked on top of one another. Sometimes, those decisions lead you to a wall that you can't get around. What do you do? You turn around and find a different path (or you smash through the wall like Koolaid Man...who is my spirit animal). You learn, you adapt, you move on.

You'll never please everyone. You'll never get the same validation from everyone. At the end of the day, it comes down to you. I know you want to please people, we all do. No one wants to stir the water or make people unhappy. But leaders have to make the tough decision and we know that people will always have their own opinion. You just can't please everyone, it's just how it goes.

I can't tell you how long it should take to make a decision or that all decisions will work out the way you think they will. I will tell you that nothing will change if you do nothing.

You control your actions, your emotions, your beliefs, your attitude. Don't get paralyzed and do nothing, life is far too short for that. You're a leader, and leaders lead. People don't follow leaders for long that don't have a direction, but rather they follow ones that have a solid foundation and know themselves. This is your world, your kingdom, you're the queen. You get to make the moves, you also are responsible for them. Move forward in confidence. Don't be afraid to pick a path. Be your CEO and lead yourself where you want to go.

You got this!

"You are only one decision from a totally different life."

-Anonymous

Chapter 14: Are You a Bazaar or a Store? Know Your Value.

I think most of us are our own worst critics. I know I was. I would look in the mirror and make a nasty face if I didn't think I looked good. I would get critical and negative with myself if I didn't do something well enough. I would criticize myself quite often.

I definitely was not asking myself if this way of thinking was serving me.

How does it serve you to tear yourself down?

What are you saying about your value?

Let's say you worked in sales. Every try to sell a product you didn't believe in? You go out into the market to sell a product and tell people it's average, could be better, doesn't look great. Do you think people would buy from you?

The way you present a product matters. If you are not confident, if you don't see the value in what you're offering, then it's going to be real hard for anyone else to want to buy.

If you walk into a store and ask for a recommendation, you expect a level of knowledge and certainty. If the store attendant isn't sure, then do you really want to spend your money on a product that might not work for you? You want confidence when you buy. You want confidence in knowing the product is going to be the right one for you. You want confidence in the quality. You want confidence where you put your money.

I was my own worst enemy and my biggest critic. I could find every reason why I wasn't perfect and why I wasn't good enough. Other people could pay me compliments, but in my mind, I rejected most of them.

What I never understood was the impact the inside of me had on the outside. I didn't understand that our value, happiness, success was all an inside job. Whatever is happening internally will impact the external. If you don't believe in yourself then what is propelling you to make it happen? If you don't believe you're smart enough to figure something out then why would you try? If you don't think you're worthy of being loved then are attracting the right person to love you? The outside is a reflection of the inside; the two are not independent of one another.

If you want to be valued then you need to have value on the inside. If you want to be loved then you need to have love on the inside. If you want happiness then you need happiness on the inside. The inside will impact the external so what you say to yourself matters!

For many years, my dating life was a mess. These guys were the worst. Let's see, I had one guy I was dating and his baby's momma called me while she was still pregnant. She wanted me to know that I was dating her boyfriend. Excuse me...*what*?! Guess he forgot to mention he was in a relationship with someone who was pregnant with his child!!

Then, there was that guy who made time for all his hobbies and would give me maybe a couple of hours a week. Learning Chinese for absolutely no reason and researching exotic fish was way more important than spending time with me. And of course, he wasn't interested in my hobbies, but he allowed me to participate in some of his when it was convenient for him.

Then, there was the physically and mentally abusive narcissist. That was a huge learning experience for me and one I've definitely grown from.

Oh, and what about that guy whose parents came and did an intervention because of his meth addiction. His what?! Yep, meth addiction. I didn't know he was on meth, but you had better believe I watched every YouTube video on the stuff after I figured out what was happening! His father, who was seven feet tall (I'm not embellishing), looked down and asked me what else he was taking. OK, I had about zero clue about anything, so I am probably the least informed one in this intervention!

It's almost comical thinking through these disasters. This was my life. This was the sum total of my dating career. These were not Hallmark winning relationships, rather some Jerry Springer entertainment, at best. Although it could be easy to finger point at the pitfalls of these guys, there was one common denominator in all of these situations. That common denominator was me.

I kept attracting guys that didn't value me. I kept attracting guys that didn't treat me right. I kept attracting guys that didn't respect me.

How could this keep happening over and over?

I didn't value me. I didn't treat me right. I didn't respect me. Remember, you're like a magnet, you attract what you put out. If you want to be valued, then you need to know your value.

How you look at yourself impacts how others look at you.

It wasn't just my dating life that didn't meet my

expectations.

I was underpaid at work.

I was underutilized at work.

The guys I dated didn't value me.

I had a high ratio of friends with little substance to them.

I was attracting zero value because I didn't set my own value.

You don't walk into a Nike store and tell the owner what you want to pay. Even if you tried, that's not the way it works. The price is set. The shoes may be on sale, but you have zero say in the price. The price is set by the store, not yourself.

Now, if you go to a bazaar, sure, you're able to bargain and negotiate. There is no saying how much something will go for, it all depends how desperate the person is to sell their goods and wares. Twenty dollars for shoes may be too low if they've sold enough that day. Or that may sound reasonable if they haven't sold anything. You have every right to negotiate at a bazaar, sellers expect this from their buyers.

I was a bazaar, not a store. I allowed the company to set my price. I allowed the company to determine my job. I allowed the guys to treat me like crap. I brought friends into my life that didn't have a depth or value to themselves.

[Side note, those who gossip to you, will gossip about you. I learned that lesson. Choose your circle wisely.]

I didn't set a price for me to be the employee. I didn't set the standard for what job I was willing to take. I didn't set the bar for how I should be treated. I didn't stop to think what kind of friends I wanted in my life. The world chose for me because I didn't.

When I figured out I was the problem and needed to fix myself from the inside out- I got on that like white on rice! It was time for me to set my value and show the world how I was to be treated.

Finding self-worth and value won't happen overnight, it's an evolution. I had to get honest with myself and stop being my worst enemy. I needed to show kindness, compassion, and care for the woman in the mirror. I needed to love of her in the way I would honor and respect a relationship with someone else.

My methodology, Date Yourself™, is based off my own journey. I connected with myself by treating me like I would any new relationship. I learned what I liked, didn't like, my strengths, my weaknesses, I did nice things for myself, I went on dates by myself, I spent time honoring and appreciating this new relationship. I fell in love with me and I found self-worth and my value in the process.

I was now able to see what I brought to the table. I celebrated me instead of tearing me down. I was the cheerleader instead of the person with a whip telling myself that I could do better. I treated myself like someone I loved, or my cat. When I began to see myself for who I was then it wasn't a question if I would accept less. I set the price.

Your self-image is created from beliefs of the past. You know you own your beliefs so change them if they don't serve you!

Watch how you talk to yourself. How you talk to yourself anytime is how you'll show up all the time. Where your thoughts go your energy flows. If you are sending signals to your brain that:

- you suck
- you're not good enough
- you're not pretty enough
- you're not worth the raise
- you don't deserve the praise
- you don't have a say in how people treat you
- your opinion doesn't matter
- you're flawed
- your personality is boring or too big
- you're not good enough to date

then remember, your brain will find reasons to believe these are true. Lead your brain where it should go.

In addition to knowing your value, take accountability

for everything that happens in your life. It's easy to blame people and situations and things that happen. It's much harder to look for your own responsibility in the situation. This game of life isn't a *who's at fault* game, but rather a game of results. Blaming and deferring accountability doesn't make forward progress.

Your biological clock isn't stopping, how much time do you want to waste pointing fingers at others and making slow to no forward momentum. I don't agree with how any of these guys treated me, but I saw that I had responsibility in the situation and I needed to be accountable for the change. When I realized this, I made the appropriate changes to ensure it didn't happen again. I was the only way out of the vicious dating cycle; my value needed to be defined.

You are the common denominator in your life and the only one responsible for the outcome. Period.

Taking accountability is the only way you are going to become your own CEO and lead your life. The CEO would get fired if excuses were made. They are to provide leadership, solutions, and results. Not excuses. Not blame. You're the CEO, this is your game of life. Set your value. When you set your value then people aren't going to haggle you. You're going to get more of what you want and not leave life to chance. People will be able to see a quality product that they'll be more inclined to invest in.

~~~

Confidence comes from within. Confidence is self-love, it's knowing yourself, it's setting your value. You are an ecosystem and all parts of how you are made up matter. When you come from a place of abundance then you won't fill voids with desperation or negativity. Love will fill your soul and when you know your value, you won't have to take just anything that comes along.

I've known plenty of women who want so desperately to be in a relationship. I was once one of these women, so it's not unfamiliar. Happiness will only come when you're in a relationship, right?

Wrong.

Everything in your life should be a compliment to what you already have. Seek to be the full sponge. When something comes along your way that compliments your life then it's a bonus.

Everything you do matters!

What you feed yourself matters.

What you listen to matters.

Who you surround yourself with matters.

How you invest your time matters.

How you talk to and value yourself matters!

It all matters!

And, when you're filled with the right ingredients-
you've discovered the recipe for a beautiful life.

There's a reason Mrs. Field's Cookies recipe is worth
450 million dollars. Every ingredient is just the right
amount and complimentary to the other. Your
ingredients matter.

It literally starts with you! Yes, you can get confident by
practicing, by being positive, by eliminating the idea of
failure, and by stopping yourself from comparing
yourself to others. But if you don't love and respect
who you are- then you're missing the most important
ingredient of the recipe.

You can make the choice today to change the way you
think about yourself.

You can make the choice today to change the way you
talk to yourself.

You can make the choice today to place a value on how
much you're worth.

You can make the choice today to become your biggest
advocate instead of your biggest enemy.

You can make the choice today to change the way you
show up in the world; powerfully over desperately.

You can make the choice today to choose to be enough

just as you are.

You can make the choice today to be beautiful just as you are.

You can make the choice today to be the most amazing support system you'll ever have.

You can make the choice today to choose love over hate, because hate breeds negativity and that polarizes confidence.

You own all these choices. You own your value. You own your happiness. You own your confidence. You own the outcome.

Make the choice.

Choose you.

Are you a bazaar or a store? If you haven't decided, then someone else will.

PS- I love you.

"Love yourself first and everything else falls into line. You really have to love yourself to get anything done in this world."

- Lucille Ball

Chapter 15: Road Blocked? Now What?

Warning, Warning,
Turn around or drown

Funny. Not funny. But Texas has these signs on the highway to get your attention! Although it's rare we have *that* much rain here in this great state, but I have seen flooding.

We know that confidence is the belief in yourself and your abilities. But what happens when you're going through life and there's a sign that says *turn around or drown*. You have full confidence that you are going to succeed, you know everything is going to be OK, but you just took a major pivot. Now what?

Roadblocks can be a trap for your confidence. You

believe in you, but the universe had a different plan.

I've often said that God won't give you more than you can handle, and clearly- He thinks I'm a rock star! I believe this because I've had so many roadblocks in my life that could have taken me down, and yet I kept getting back in the game.

So, what do you do when you run into what looks like a stopping point? How do you remain confident when it looks like not everything is OK?

You find the opportunity.

So, the business didn't turn out the way you thought it would. No one bought the course you spent time and money to create. Your relationship fell apart. You got laid off. Your friends turned out to be different than you thought they were. Maybe you got diagnosed with an illness. These can all look like roadblocks. When they happen, it's easier to be like a turtle and hide in your shell.

I know a woman, a beautiful woman, that used to work for one of the most well-known modeling agencies. She modeled all over the world, including Milan, Italy, one of the most prestigious places to walk on a runway. Although not overly noticeable, I could tell she had some work done on her nose. I never asked her what happened or why it appeared to look a little different, but I had some curiosity.

One day, she shared her journey with me. She said she was so immersed in her fame and beauty that she listened to someone's suggestion for her to get some work done on her nose. Looking at pictures I saw no need for this work, but beauty is in the eye of the beholder. She went to get her nose worked on and to her dismay, too much cartilage was taken out. Her nose collapsed.

If there was ever a roadblock, this certainly could have been one. My heart felt for her as I listened to her share her story. With a humbleness about her, she told me how she had undergone countless surgeries to correct the mistake and reverse the procedure. She had upward of twenty to thirty surgeries, and still there were signs work had been done.

Imagine being in her shoes. Imagine having a life that little girls dream about; being a model, working in Italy, having beauty that catches everyone's attention. With one decision, your life changes overnight. Her career as she knew it came to a halt.

I wanted to hug her as I listened, my heart felt her story. Then, the real beauty inside her surfaced.

I felt gratitude from my friend for what had happened in her life. Although she didn't want her nose to collapse, it allowed her to reconnect with herself and tap into areas where she could be of service to others. She found talents and skills she didn't know existed, and now she helps other women feel and look their best.

When I see my friend, I see strength and courage. It's much easier to curl up and want to hide away. We can get so far into our heads of what other people may think. We care what others will say, the stories people will make up, the judgements, the finger pointing. When roadblocks occur, they can come in any shape and size, and they can damage our confidence.

This is when you need to take control in your mind. An uncontrolled mind can play games and tricks and make you think the world is against you. An uncontrolled mind may make you feel like a failure. It can take the wind out of your sail and make you think you're not good enough. You need to ensure yourself that everything is going to be OK. Own your dialogue, don't let it own you.

When my friend encountered a new face, which resulted in a change in her career, it wasn't a dead-end. Rather, she found freedom to reinvent herself. She found hope and peace in knowing she could help others through her journey. She chose to find strength over defeat. She was not a victim, but rather found the opportunity to grow and connect with her most powerful self.

What is opportunity?

Freedom. Hope. Shot. Fortuity.

The opposite of opportunity?

Closure. Misfortune. Dead-end. Pitfall.

Which sounds more like where you want to align? Is the world ending or just beginning for you?

When we're focused on opportunity- we have a goal. When we're working towards a goal- we have purpose. When we have purpose then our life has meaning. Remember, as Zig Ziglar said, "if you aim at nothing, you hit your target every time." When we encounter a roadblock, it can stop us in our tracks. We sometimes lose sight of the goal. We lose the confidence we had that propelled us to that point.

One of my jobs in corporate really stands out to me. This job was full of opportunity. I could have chosen to look at it as a disaster, but I chose to find the potential and the abundant room for growth. The truth was, this company had so many holes and gaps. It lacked structure. It lacked processes. The leadership lacked innovation and it was trying to squeeze lemon juice from a turnip. I very easily could have locked at this as a sinking ship and dysfunctional mess, but the idea of opportunity excited me.

Imagine being in a tech company and yet leadership doesn't want to adopt electronic signatures. Instead, they're more comfortable with physical signatures. This meant we would have to physically run around and get five levels of authorized signatures to sign a contract.

I'm sorry, is it 1960? Why on earth would we be physically running around in 2019 getting physical signatures? Oh, because you trust ink on paper more than you do DocuSign, the same technology you probably used to buy your house? Hum. Sure, that makes sense (sense my sarcasm?)!

As insane as this archaic habit was, I saw it as opportunity. I tasked my team with spearheading automation, knowing this would be an uphill battle. It wasn't easy, but my team was successful in implementing this process change.

Whenever I hired staff for that company, it was important for me to understand how the candidates viewed roadblocks. If they saw opportunity, then they scored higher in their interviews. Knowing the company had landmines and challenges in every direction, I needed to have staff who could look beyond the surface level to innovate and drive new solutions.

Opportunity is potential, it's possibilities, it's limitless!

There is always more than one way to look at a situation. You may only see one option on the surface. This roadblock may look like a closed door. But here is your opportunity to have a choice mindset rather than seeing no other options.

Opportunity doesn't always present itself on a pretty platter. If it did, I think we might miss a lot of opportunities. We might not even notice them because they wouldn't catch our attention. I honestly believe that most lessons and opportunities come when life gets shaken up. You know, like the martini you order? Yes, shaken, not stirred, that's where you'll find lessons and opportunities.

Think about when that door appeared to get slammed in your face. That was an opportunity.

Think about the time that a situation went seriously south. That was an opportunity.

Thank about a time when you thought there was no hope and your back was against a wall. That was an opportunity.

Think about my friend that went through a traumatic surgery. That was an opportunity.

When you see that rotting, smelly, dumpster fire; that's opportunity!

I interviewed an incredible woman and past Olympian, Kelly Gunther, for the *Level Up To 2.0* podcast. To say I was blown away by the positivity and confidence from this woman would be an understatement. Although Kelly grew up with learning disabilities, she never let that stop her. The first time she saw a figure skater, she knew that she wanted to be an Olympic skater. She had never so much as set foot on ice, but she wasn't going to let that stop her.

Kelly already had dreams and the only thing she saw was opportunity. Why not her? There was no fathomable reason why she shouldn't be the one to represent her country.

And that's what Kelly set out to do, she was going to be in the Olympics. First roadblock, she didn't know how to skate. Practice. Practice. Practice. Kelly practiced her heart out.

Next roadblock. She couldn't hear the music well enough to stay on rhythm. How was she ever going to be able to perform a routine if she couldn't hear well?

But Kelly had a dream.

She looked for the opportunity. Speed skating.

Kelly didn't need to hear the music in order to speed skate. And, although it didn't have the same girly clothing that went along with being a figure skater, she could still be on the ice and go where most only ever dream to be, the Olympics.

There she was, now a speed skater. She sat around with her peers the day the announcements were made of who was going to be on the US Team. She sat optimistically. Her name wasn't called. Roadblock.

Kelly again looked for the opportunity. Next time, she thought.

She made the choice in her mind that she would be

more prepared next time around.

And that's what Kelly set out to do.

One day, during practice, Kelly's world changed, yet again. The horn blared and Kelly took off from the starting point on the ice. Kelly loved the thrill of hearing the horn blare and the feeling of her gliding along the ice with the blades strapped to her feet. This time was different. Kelly heard the horn and took off skating. Almost immediately, her skate got stuck, and due to the speed at which she was moving, her foot detached her body. As her body came to a stop on the ice, she told herself she was only going to look down one time.

And there it was; a skater's worst nightmare.

Roadblock.

To be a skater and lose the use of your foot could be a game changer. As I interviewed this young woman, she had a level of confidence and ease through every perceivable roadblock. What came next was the most shocking of all.

Kelly Gunther, a woman from a small town with big dreams, said injuring her foot was the best thing that ever happened to her.

It's almost unfathomable how someone can be so positive about injuring their foot. It's a choice. It's a choice how you interpret the situation. You can allow it to cripple you or strengthen you. This wasn't a stopping point for Ms. Gunther, she didn't even see this as a reason to pivot away from her dream. She made the commitment to herself to get back out there and go to the Olympics; same purpose and commitment she's always had.

One screw and 10 pins later, the doctors were able to reposition her foot back where it started. It's amazing to think how far we've come with modern medicine. This traumatic event was nothing more than moment in time that eventually healed.

Kelly is one of the most tenacious and incredible women I've had the opportunity to speak with. She's the *Comeback Kid* for a reason, because every time something in her life happened, she always made a comeback. There wasn't a question of *if*, it was a question of *when*. She went on to make the 2014 US Olympic speed skating team, and I couldn't be more proud of this young, tenacious woman.

I hope you never lose a limb. I hope your business never tanks. I hope your spouse never leaves you. I hope your surgery goes as expected. But your life *will* have outcomes you don't expect. When they arise, and they will, tap into opportunity. Don't let the world take the wind out of your sail. Stand in freedom, hope, fortuity. These are confident stances and will help you maintain footing when life may seem a little shaky.

If Kelly can find opportunity in the moment she nearly lost her foot, if my friend can find the good when her nose job failed, then any of us can train our minds to look at roadblocks and challenges as opportunities. With opportunity comes confidence. They're both a mindset, and a mindset that you can choose to propel or repel you.

Opportunity is freedom, it's hope, it's another shot. Mindset is how you choose to look at everything in your life. If roadblocks stand in your way, then it's devastating when they happen. If roadblocks open up more doors, then your world is limitless. Check your beliefs, do they serve you?

Roadblocks are opportunities, even when they look like a box that's been run over on the highway. Embrace it. Love it. Seek it. Have confidence in knowing the world is working for you if you choose to see it that way.

"If you're trying to achieve, there will be roadblocks. I've had them; everybody has had them. But obstacles don't have to stop you. If you run into a wall, don't turn around and give up. Figure out how to climb it, go through it, or work around it."

-Michael Jordan

Chapter 16: Starting Over

I hope by this point that you're tuned in to a few key points:

- The universe is working for you
- The brain is a goal achieving machine
- You can rewire your thoughts
- Where your thoughts go your energy flows
- Beliefs create experiences
- You own your beliefs
- Failure doesn't have to exist
- Everything in your life is designed to make you who you are
- Confidence is a mindset
- Mindset is everything

I believe that's about a $25K masterclass right there, so you're welcome. These are fundamental principles and keys to your success.

There is often a perspective I hear that starting over or reducing your footprint in life is taking a step back. It's the house, the cars, the bank account, the responsibilities, all should get bigger with time. If this is what you believe then you'll always be seeking more and bigger. If life throws a challenge at you and you need to downsize then you'll find yourself in a world of suffering. You get to choose what you believe, but I'm here to suggest that starting over is not a bad thing. When you are able to be in flow with your life then you'll find you have a higher degree of confidence; you disconnect emotions with the outcome.

Before I became an entrepreneur, I had a house, a large truck, and a decent enough salary. Entering into my entrepreneurial journey, I moved into the smallest apartment I had ever lived in, I sold my vehicle, and I didn't have predictable income. This could very well have looked like a step back in life if you chose it to look that way.

I want to offer a different perspective. As you move through your life, instead of focusing on size, what if you asked yourself that one powerful question we keep referring to; does this serve me?

If it doesn't serve you to have a larger house, a bigger vehicle, a larger paycheck, then why would you choose size over what makes sense for your life?

Knowing I was going to be leaving corporate, I started to

make moves around downsizing my life. I knew I was going to have unpredictable income in the beginning. I didn't want to be bothered with paying the exorbitant taxes in Dallas County and a mortgage.

I knew a lot of my free *time* was going to be focused around building my business. I didn't want to be bothered with mowing lawns, changing lightbulbs, fixing anything that broke around the house. I wanted my energy to go into building a business rather than the upkeep of a house. So, I moved. I took my cat, Booger, and we went on an adventure together into a tiny, 617 square foot apartment. There was less cleaning, less maintenance, less responsibilities. This served me more than having a house and mowing a lawn with grass that needed consistent attention.

I even decided I was going to change the way I ate because I was spending way too long in the kitchen meal prepping every week. I was accustomed to spending three to four hours cooking every Sunday and preparing meals for the week. It took far less time for me to eat precut carrots and veggie patties, so that's what I did. I gained hours back by changing the way I ate.

I also decided I was going to sell my vehicle. I had a beautiful truck, but vehicles cost money and take time. I didn't want to do oil changes, go to the car wash, pump tires, get gas, sit in traffic, or spend the money, quite frankly. When I have a vehicle, I don't think so much about where I need to go, I just get in my truck and drive. Without a vehicle, you become a lot more aware of getting from place to place. When you pay for an Uber and it costs $50, you think about the trip a bit more. I didn't need to be driving around, I needed to be building my business. I sold my truck. I'm probably the only one I know that made this commitment to building her business, but I was exceedingly happy with these decisions.

Selling my truck, selling my house, eating carrots and hummus over prepared meals may have looked like a step back. Each one of these decisions was made intentionally and I still stand behind all of them. I asked myself at every step of the way if my lifestyle or things served me. I asked myself if what I was investing my time in served me. I asked myself if where I put my thoughts served me. If something didn't, then I changed it.

I was less focused on having a plethora of material things and responsibilities. Instead, I was more focused on what was best for me at that time given the goals I wanted to achieve.

It's funny how those four words will help drive decisions that work for you in your life if you are honest with yourself.

Does this serve me?

[My hope by now is that your brain is rewired to always

default to this question since we're referenced it in almost every chapter. Repetition creates confidence!]

From the outside looking in, it very well could look like a step back. To me, I believed I made some of the smartest decisions I could have made. I chose to invest my time, energy, and resources into myself. Making this change allowed me to follow my dream.

I couldn't have been happier and more sure of the decisions made to minimize my life. In fact, I made these moves before COVID hit, and I think a lot of people may have changed their mind on how they viewed my downsizing. I had fewer bills, needed less Clorox wipes, I had more time, I could easily order groceries, the world turned virtual and that was perfect since I sold my car!

The idea that stuff or money equates to success is merely a belief. It's the same belief we talked about with my friend's father. To him, success equaled money. I chose to take another definition of success.

Whatever you choose to believe is your truth. I choose to believe that starting over is not a failure. It's not an indication on how successful you are. It's not a measure of whether or not you are a good person or not. In fact, I think it takes someone that is strong and wise to pull the plug and change direction. Change can be scary, and it keeps people from growth. It takes bravery to shift. This applies to anything in your life.

Where you live, who you're friends with, your job, your business, the kind of house you own.

Your life is going to continue to change as you age and you'll have different mindsets, different skills, different needs, different variables; life is fluid.

I think about where I was in my life when I was 16 years of age. It didn't matter how much money I made, I just needed enough for gas and clothes. It didn't matter where I lived, my parents made that decision for me. At 16, I was just coasting. Not a lot of responsibilities, just get through high school. Then, when I was 35, life looked different. It mattered how much money I made. It mattered if I had a vehicle. It mattered the kind of job I had. I wanted a salary that would substantiate buying a house, so I needed to have a job to support that lifestyle. When I'm 70, I hope I'm retired. I hope that along the way I've saved money because I probably won't want to work at that point. I probably won't want to take care of a house either.

At every point in your life is going to look different. Life needs to fit you. Don't let society make decisions for you about what you should or should not be doing, you are in the driver's seat. Watch out for living someone else's dream of success. Be the one to own the choices in your life, even if looks like you are starting over.

Have you ever put too much of an ingredient in something you're making? Maybe you're making cookies and instead of two cups of sugar, you put in two cups of salt. Imagine what that would taste like. You could just bake the cookies as they are, but I guarantee they're going to be like a salt-lick to eat. Or you could modify the recipe and keep adding the other ingredients and make a *really large* batch of cookies to equal out the salt. That's certainly an option. Or you could start over.

Starting over isn't a bad thing, it's an opportunity.

It's an opportunity to do something different.

It's an opportunity to do something better.

It's an opportunity to get rid of the gunk and rebuild with a fresh slate.

It takes a confident person to start over and know that it will be OK. It's the trust that you're making the right decisions. It's faith that the world is working for you. Honestly, I think it takes courage, it shows strength. You've opted to start from scratch vs. bandaiding something together.

For you, it might be:

- ending a relationship that was over years ago
- leaving corporate and stepping into the entrepreneurial space
- building the next business
- creating a new product line

- changing your friends
- moving to a new city
- downsizing to an apartment
- exploring a new religion
- changing the way you eat
- changing your look
- throwing out that batter and starting from scratch

There are loads of ways that you might find you need to start over, and I'm here to tell you that it's OK. Your view on starting over is a belief; don't allow it scare you and steal your confidence.

Perfection doesn't exist. Not one of us on this earth walked a perfect life, except Jesus. If people are expecting perfection out of you then is that really the circle you want to be spending your time in? A perfect life is a belief, it's an idea, it's not a fact.

At the end of the day, you are the only one that needs to be concerned with your thoughts, your actions, your life. You are the sole owner of your happiness, your success, your actions, your emotions, and what you get out of life. Aim for this idea of successful versus success. How might that change your perception?

Starting over is failure if you believe it to be. I believe it's courageous and sometimes necessary. I think it's braver to do than sticking with what you have, it says a lot about your character.

Don't think you're stuck with salty batter, you never are. You learn, you course correct, you grow. It is always OK to start over, just focus on you. And, if that batter is still salty-- try again! Be confident in knowing that you own the keys to your kingdom and you define how it looks.

As Zen Cho said, "If at first you don't succeed, try, try again."

"Though nobody can go back and make a new beginning, anyone can start over and make a new ending."

— Chico Xavier

Chapter 17: Surrounded by Confidence

"You become like the five people you spend the most time with. Choose carefully."

-Jim Rohn

Imagine you want to start a business. You have this idea for a product that doesn't exist in the market and you are convinced it's a multi-million dollar idea. You've been dreaming about the potential and you can't get it out of your head.

You start to tell your friends. First, your best friend.

"Girl, I have this idea, you aren't going to believe it!"

You tell her all the details and she looks at you and says, "You're crazy."

Ouch, not entirely the response you were looking for.

But that's OK. She tried building a business once and lost a bunch of money so you understand why she may be a little jaded.

You have lunch with the girls a few weeks later and you tell them of your idea. Now, you're really confident in your idea, you've thought through every little detail and it's perfect!

You tell the girls, and then….crickets.

"Sounds pretty risky."

"What do your parents think?"

"Did you talk to an expert?"

"What if it fails?"

Wow, more negative responses you didn't see coming. You change the subject; you don't even want to talk about it anymore. Last stop; mom and dad.

"I don't know, honey, we want the best for you, don't you think that's a lot work and scary? What if people don't like it and you've wasted all this money?"

You start to question your idea. Maybe it's not the best idea and maybe it will only lead to failure. What then?! You run through your idea over and over and now, all you can think about is how hard it's going to be and how you'll have to give up your security of corporate to pursue this wild idea. Probably good to stop before getting started, right?

Your idea got shot down, it's no surprise you decided to give up on the dream. Even though you saw the potential and thought through every situation, you gave up your dream because no one else saw it. It's not always easy being the lone ranger pioneering through the dark forest. No one gave you a glimmer of hope or a sign of support. It's not too surprising you changed your mind.

What if, when you told your mentor about your idea that she said, "You're on to something. Chase it!"

How would that feel?

Then, you go to the luncheon of likeminded individuals and you make the announcement feeling pretty good about the fact that your mentor loved the idea. You deliver the idea with such energy and excitement, you're optimistic they'll love the idea too! And they were!

"That's genius!"

"How can we support you?"

"Your parents are going to be so proud!"

"We've got investors you should talk to."

More affirmation. It's like landing in a security blanket. Your network is on board with supporting you and encouraging you, and it feels really darn good.

How differently does it feel to have support? Makes you more confident, doesn't it? When you're around people that understand your journey, that are on similar paths, that have your best interest at heart it will boost your confidence. There's not just power in numbers, but confidence in numbers. Many people will not understand your journey, and that's OK, but there are plenty of people out there that will.

If it's for support for your business, religion, mindset, parental support, whatever is relevant in your life, it's important you surround yourself with likeminded individuals. When you approach these people with your ideas, your challenges, your opportunities, then you'll be able to get sound advice. If someone doesn't know how to relate to your journey, then it's hard for them to know how to empathize and advise.

It's not the responsibility of your family and close friends to support you in the capacity you need, but rather it's your responsibility to find the people that are going to relate and understand your journey. Find the people that are able to support you and have conversations appropriately. This doesn't mean to get rid of family and close friends, it just means you need to have the awareness of who to talk to and where to get support.

This group will be your go-to when you have questions,

need community, or want to share your wins. When it looks like life became dismal, they can help talk you through it. When you have an idea, they can be a sounding board. You'll get advice that doesn't falsely elevate or reject your idea, but rather real advice from people that have been there. They can celebrate in your success and understand the journey it took to get there. These are your people!

Maybe you went through a miscarriage, had a heart attack, moved abroad, started a business, got laid off, got divorced, got cheated on, had a child with a rare genetic disorder, had a child that wanted to transition their sex, got engaged, whatever it is, it's your responsibility to find the support you need. When you do, your confidence will elevate.

Imagine you get engaged? You'll probably find a wedding planner, contact a venue, call your girlfriends that just got married. You'll call someone that knows about weddings. You can certainly elicit help from your unmarried friends that have no experience, but does that give you the level of confidence you need going into your own wedding. You may decide you don't want an expert to help, and you're fine with having friends that have never planned or been in a wedding coordinate the logistics. That's a risk that you assume. It's not the responsibility of your friends with no experience to be the experts. They will do the best they can, but it's a decision you chose and the risk you need to be willing to make. Remember, you take full responsibility for the decisions you make in your life. If you want confidence in your wedding, then you need to find the right people to support you.

One of the areas I saw a gap in my life when I became an entrepreneur was having people around me that understood what I was going through. I needed more people to add intellectual value and support in my life. No fault to my current set of friends, I was just entering new territory. When you level up, you are moving from one place in your life to another. Your mind, your friends, the way you manage a business, the way you see yourself, the way you budget, and who you surround yourself with changes. You can't expect change to happen without any changes to yourself, your surroundings, the way you show up.

I found a few groups that could support me in the capacity I needed. It made all the difference. I didn't feel alone. I saw others going through similar challenges. I was able to get advice. I had people that could talk me off a ledge. I was able to share wins and not feel like I was bragging. All *ships rise with the tide,* right? There is power in numbers, you don't have to walk this life alone. Someone has gone through what you're going through. Find your people.

The right people in your space matters. It can make the difference between you starting or abandoning your dream.

It's the old adage *you are what you eat.* What you put into your mind, your body, your energy matters, it all has an impact on who you are, how you feel, and what you do with your life.

If you are surrounded by all people that like to sit around and drink beer, you may find yourself doing this rather than taking a run or working out. If you're around people that gossip, you're likely to get pulled into gossiping. If you hang out with coworkers that despise the company, then you'll likely also have a distaste for the company.

I'd encourage you to become part of a network that aligns with where you're at or where you're going. Maybe it's a women's group, a business coaching program, a social networking group, a sports league, a religious organization, a mastermind. Find a group where you align with the mission, vision, and values. Having this group to turn to for support will be instrumental in boosting your confidence and giving you the backing you need as you grow.

~~~

I took a trip with some women to Mexico and there were two of us that really enjoyed going out and dancing. We were two very tall, strong, confident women that loved getting out on a dancefloor and grooving to music. There was another woman that also came out with us, but she was more timid in her demeanor. The three of us went out and had a blast. If we were dancing by ourselves or with other people, we were having an incredible time just enjoying the moment! I'm sure all eyes were on us too because it was hard to miss these tall, beautiful, confident women (and we went on multiple stages- so there's that). At the end of the night, we went back to the hotel and ordered food. We reminisced about the evening and talked about the fun we had.

The more timid woman was especially ecstatic about the evening. She loved dancing but admitted she didn't do it often. She told us that she fed off our confidence and that helped her to let loose and dance without reservation. It was something she had inside her but didn't typically have the confidence within herself to do.

Confidence is infectious. You will draw energy from other confident people. Find them and build the faith, the trust, the belief in yourself. We learn by example and we draw strength from others.

It can be intimidating to get out of your comfort zone, to stretch yourself to the next level, to be vulnerable with the world. You may want to have the confidence to do something, but fear gets in the way. Being around other confident people and people that are on your level will help you on your journey. When you see that other people can do what you're set out to do and they survive, it gives you tangible examples that the world won't fall apart if you give it a try. When you have people cheering you on, it's easier to believe in yourself too.

~~~

Be who you want to be surrounded by and choose a circle of people you want to be like. Since like attracts like, be aware of your own energy and mindset you put out in the world. Like a boomerang, what you put out will come back.

Have you ever met someone that's negative and loving life? It's like oil and water, they don't mix. If you're positive, it's a breeding ground for joy and peace. If you're negative, it's a breeding ground for misery. The energy you choose to be around and have within you is going to have an impact on your experience in life.

Think of someone that's negative all the time. You know, that Negative Nancy, Debbie Downer or the Karen's of this world (why are there no negative men that we use in these examples….there's also that Chatty Cathy…hummmmm). Think of that person. It's a lot to be around them and you can take them in only small doses. Why? Because it's soul sucking. Imagine what it's like to be that person. Even if an opportunity presented itself, that person would have a hard time seeing it because there'd be some negative spin they'd fixate on. Doesn't matter if it's the perfect temperature and no clouds outside, there'd be some reason to be negative.

Ever met someone that laughs so much that you can't help but laugh too? Or someone that has so much self-love that it starts to rub off? I was watching a YouTube video the other day and this 22-year-old woman, Michelle, had a rare genetic disorder. Michelle was one of only a few hundred cases to have Hallerman-Streiff syndrome. From the outside, she was unlike anyone I had ever seen. She had 26 of the 28 genetic characteristics that make up this rare disorder. It was very noticeable by her appearance that she was physically different than other people. This woman had more self-love than probably 99% of people in this world. She loved everything about herself. I'm certain she's faced adversity, heard cruel comments, and been shunned by people. In no way do I imagine this woman has had it easy, and yet, she had the most self-love of almost anyone I've seen.

Michelle didn't compare herself to others, she embraced who she was. She loved the person she saw in the mirror and wasn't going to be defined by anyone other than herself. Her family was in the interview with her and it was clear she had an incredible support system of love. Although they admitted it had its challenges and difficulties, they also said loving this woman was the greatest gift they could have ever imagined. It helped to give them a perspective on self-love and loving people for who they are and are not. Michelle's self-love was able to impact her family in how they experienced love in their own lives.

Although I have a lot of self-love and self-confidence, it's hard not to be moved by Michelle's story. If she can love herself with all the challenges she faces, then who am I to judge myself for any of my imperfections. If she can get up and be positive even though she has a tube in her throat and can barely see, then what do I have to complain about in my life that is pretty normal? Her energy and positivity was so infectious. If we could bottle it up and sell it then this world would be a drastically different place.

Energy is magnetic. From the inside out, the energy in your space matters.

I'd encourage you to assess yourself. Do you think you're a negative or a positive person? If you truly don't know or aren't sure, go ask someone whom you respect and that you believe to be positive. You might not even realize the negativity you carry within you.

I remember when I was dating this guy, I would send him little videos every morning on my way into work. When we broke up, I started to do a lot of personal development work and I found myself on a general quest for happiness. After a few months, I decided to go back and look at some of those videos. I was shocked. I thought I was sending sweet videos. What I saw with my new positive outlook on life was quite the opposite. There was always some underpinning of negativity in all the videos! Maybe a train would pass by and I would be expressing my annoyance by the inconvenience it caused my life. Or maybe I felt the need to talk about the lack of sleep I got. Or maybe I needed to talk about how I wasn't excited to go to work. Whatever it was, I was much more negative than I realized. This was the same guy that told me I needed to learn to love myself. It was evident to him that I was hurting and it wasn't the right energy for him. I applaud him for making the decision to protect his own energy.

There's a phenomenon when you start to get rid of negativity in your life. You'll find that you have little to no tolerance for energy that weighs you down. As you let go of the past, stop being around gossip, disassociate with the nay-sayers, you'll feel the difference and reject it when it comes into your space.

Positivity, like confidence, is a mindset. It's a choice you make. And when you choose to be positive, life isn't overwhelming when it doesn't turn out the way you think it will. You'll be able to look at your life and find the good in the bad. You'll be like Michelle and focus on every good thing about yourself. You'll have more confidence to try new things because you won't be focused on a potentially negative outcome. Life is different when you show up positively. Being around positive people is going to help lift you up. Conversely, negativity will hold you back.

Confidence is positivity. Keeping a confident mindset and surrounding yourself with confident people will elevate you on your journey.

At the end of the day, it's you that needs to believe in yourself. You need to have the confidence in your vision, skills, abilities, otherwise you'll fall off the bull before the gate opens and the rodeo begins. You need to have trust, faith, and belief that what you are doing is the right thing. The people you surround yourself with can help your journey. Find the ones that are aligned with where you want to be, want to support you, and exhibit the confidence you want in your own life. Be mindful of your energy. Be that magnetic force of positivity and radiance and you'll see the brilliance of what you attract!

"If you surround yourself with positive people who build you up, the sky is the limit."

-Joel Brown

Chapter 18: Showing Up with Confidence

Shoulder back, chin up, and wipe those tears away!

Sounds like the advice your parents gave you after crashing your bike into a tree, doesn't it (I would know, I crashed into a few).

Although confidence is an inside job, there are things you can do to help look and feel confident on the outside. Confidence is made to be seen, not bottled up and hid, so let's get your outside shining like the inside to really get noticed.

I had a guy reach out to me recently to be a guest on my podcast, *Level Up To 2.0*. I'm pretty selective with whom I bring on the show and I tend to be booked pretty far in advance. There was something, however, that I couldn't ignore about his energy; it was powerful, and I said yes without reservation.

He created a program that changed his life in such a positive way that he was on fire to share it with the world! He sent me a message through Facebook. When I heard it, I was intrigued to learn more because he brought so much energy and enthusiasm to what he was offering. He had confidence in his product, and I heard it through his voice.

It was clear that he believed in what he was doing. Not in a cocky or inauthentic way, but rather in a genuine sense because of how it changed his life. Had I just come across his page and seen his program then it may not have caught my attention. How he put himself out there and confidently connected with me was what made me intrigued to learn more.

It's one thing to have internal confidence, but if you just keep it to yourself- will you be achieving all your goals?

You want to get in a relationship- you need to be seen.

You want to start a business- you need to be seen.

You're selling something- you need to be seen.

You want a new job- you need to be seen.

You want to find a new tribe- you need to be seen.

You want to participate in your kid's school- you need to be seen.

You want to volunteer- you need to be seen.

You've built your confidence on the inside. Now how do you get the outside to match what's happening on the inside? First, you have to be willing to be seen. If you think people are just going to find you sitting in your house, news flash- that's probably not going to happen.

How do you get seen?

You need to show up where your people are going to be! If you're selling something, where does your ideal client hangout? If you want to date, where would a potential suitor be found? If you want to change jobs, where are jobs posted or who can you talk to?

People aren't mind readers. We don't find your thoughts; we find what you put out there! Showing up could be on social media, on an app, at networking events, at galas, at PTA meetings, at conferences, at the bar, at social events- there are loads of ways to show up in the world! You can start blogging! You don't even have to show your face, but you have to show something!

When you start to communicate your message- remember that everything will turn out alright and the world won't fall apart! If you approach someone to dance with you and they say NO- the world isn't going to end. If you have an idea you pitch to someone and it's not for them, then it's meant for someone else. If you apply for a job and they don't pick you, the universe probably just saved you from something that you didn't see coming. Whatever it is, the world is not going to fall apart so speak into what you want and stand behind it!

Use words that are confident- don't waiver!

The words you use matter! If the gentleman that approached me to be on my podcast said he *thought* his program would work, then I wouldn't have been interested in any more conversation. Using words like *think* and *probably* are not strong words to enforce whatever it is you're set out to do.

As a consumer, I want to know if something is going to work. I don't want *maybe*, I want certainty. Is it the best? Will the solution fulfill my need? Is it quality? Watch out for words that diminish your credibility.

- Sort of
- Maybe
- Kind of
- I think it will
- I'm pretty sure it will
- Probably is going to

Start to pay attention when you use these words and remove them as you start to notice them. This will help you show up more powerfully.

Tone matters!

If that gentleman had used a soft voice, then I probably

wouldn't have had a lot of confidence in him. I also may have dismissed it if he was monotone. I most definitely would have dismissed him if he sounded scared or his voice was cracking.

Tone matters!

People will hear the confidence in your voice and it comes through in how you present yourself. Be mindful of the tone; not too aggressive and not too soft. Use inflections when you talk, it makes it easier for people to follow along (they won't want to fall asleep). Don't sound like you're going through puberty—know your stuff! Practice and it will become more natural. Allow the words to flow through you, don't force them. You know your stuff; don't overthink.

Your physical presence matters!

Envision what someone without confidence looks like. The person in your mind may have slumped shoulders, their head down, avoid eye contact. It may even look like the person was sad, had a bad day, or was defeated. There's a solemn vibe you get as this person walks into the room (or maybe it's a zoom call since we're in a virtual world these days). How do you feel when you see this person? Is this someone you'd invest in? Is this someone you'd want to hire, do business with, date, be friends with?

Maybe.

I remember I used to cross my arms over my body because I was uncomfortable with myself. My best friend growing up told me the first time she saw me she thought I was cocky. By closing myself off, it gave the impression that I didn't want to talk to anyone. Truth was, I was insecure about myself, but that wasn't the vibe I gave off. Your stance matters. Open yourself up so people feel they can approach you. Shoulders back and arms by your side will be a much more inviting and trusting stance.

Eye contact is another powerful non-verbal form of communication. When you are willing to look someone in the eye then you are making a deeper connection with them. This can be uncomfortable for people and can take practice. But we know that practice makes you more confident, so start to become aware of looking people in the eyes when you're talk to them.

Watch the fidgeting! Imagine you're in a meeting with someone and they're playing with their hair or playing with one of those fidget spinners that got popular for like a week. Would you feel like they were connected with you or that they were distracted? Would you feel they were confident, or they were nervous and needed to channel their energy? Fidgeting isn't going to give off the confidence, connection, or the energy you want to give. Be mindful if you're playing with something- even if it's just change in your pocket!

Body language matters. When you put yourself out

there, you don't want people to think you're afraid, sad, or scared. You want someone to be drawn to your awesomeness! Confidence is positivity and it's magnetic. Open yourself up to the world. Put your shoulders back, head up, and don't be afraid to look at people in the eye. Let them see you, you're a magnificent human!

Walk with intention!

There's a noticeable difference between the person that knows where they're going and the person that looks around to figure out where they're supposed to be. Confidence doesn't always mean you know where you're going, but you can still walk with intent even when you don't!

I prefer to know where I'm headed. If I'm meeting friends in a restaurant, I usually ask them where they're at before I get there. This way, I'm not walking around aimlessly looking for them. If I genuinely don't know where my party is at, I'll still walk with conviction like I know where I'm going.   I don't have the look on my face like I'm lost, I look like I'm on a mission. You're less likely to get asked if you need help if you look like you know where you're going. It's the energy you give off, so learn to walk with intention (also be humble enough to ask when you need to, I'm not advocating arrogance and egotism).

Do what makes you feel good!

Doesn't matter to me what you wear or how you look but feel good about whatever you choose! There are different pieces of clothing I'll wear when I need that extra motivation. Depending on what I'm doing, who I'll be seeing, or where I'm going, I'll pick an outfit that I feel good about wearing.

It's important to feel confident in the clothes you're in. When you feel like you'd rather be wearing a garbage bag on your head then you aren't going to show up as powerfully! If I feel bloated, I'm not going to wear a tight shirt. If my hair is doing something weird, I'll wear it up. If my outfit lacks color, then I'll throw on a pair of colorful pumps. I make decisions that are going to make me feel good.

Whatever it is for you, focus feeling confident. If it's your hair, nails, shoes, socks, underwear, jewelry, whatever it might be—have it compliment that awesome interior.

Don't be afraid to stand out!

I have literally built my brand and my identity on the fact that I'm 6'1" and wear heels. When I walk in a room-- you can't miss me. I always tell new people I'm meeting how to find me because I don't go unnoticed. Without fail, people will confidently walk right up to me and say hello. There's no way you can miss or mistake the only woman that is 6'5"! I own it, embrace it, and I use it to my advantage. I rarely ever need to find other people; they can easily spot me!

You may not be my size, but don't afraid to share who you are with the world and let that be your identifier. The thing about you that make you unique is your special sauce. Don't dilute it, promote it! People will love you for owning those things about you that make you unique. Confidence is authenticity—let it be seen! If you have a gap in your teeth, if you have a mole on your nose, if you wear a three-piece suit-- own it!

A friend of mine, Brian, always wears a three-piece suit to a conference. I think jeans are more the norm than the exception these days, and yet Brian still wears his suits! I admire this about him and I think it makes him unique. As a society, we've moved away from formal attire. Google started allowing their employees to wear shorts to the office five-days a week and much of the world followed. Not Brian. I hope he continues to show up in his three-piece suits; it makes him unique, and I can easily spot him.

Show what you want to be seen and this is what people will remember. This goes for bad and off-putting habits as well. Remember, first impressions are key, so come out as the person you want to be known for.

Whatever it is for you-- own it! If you like wearing a neon earrings, do it! If you want an afro-- rock it! If you snort when you laugh-- own it! If you have a big personality-- be it! Be you. Be proud of that person and don't dull your shine.

There is something about you that makes you unique and you're amazing just as you are. The world needs more light! Shine brightly! Don't be afraid to stand out, it's what makes you special and will get people's attention (make sure you're focused on the right kind of attention)!

Show up visibly confident and you'll catch attention. Then hit them with the 1-2 punch and show them from the inside what you got. Confidence comes from within, but you can definitely set yourself apart by showing it on the outside. The truth is, it takes internal confidence to show outwardly that you're confident with who you are. It took me finding self-confidence to step out with 4" heels, I couldn't have done that without doing the internal work. You make a statement about your internal confidence by showing up as yourself without any apology!

What people see and hear on the outside is what will help catch their attention. You have to show up in order to be seen, so help attract the right visibility to you by making sure you're exterior and vocals match the confident mindset you've developed.

Confidence is a mindset, it's a state of being. The world needs what you have to offer. Show them what you got! And yes, confidence is sexy. Sharing it proudly will take you from a 10 to an 11 on the sexy scale! Now, go play *Sexy and I Know It* by LMFAO and practice that strut!

"No matter what a woman looks like, if she's confident, she's sexy."

-Paris Hilton

Chapter 19: Go Be the Queen

Understanding that everything you need is already inside of you is like tapping into a wishing well. You lack nothing. You get to choose your beliefs, your experiences, how you show up in the world. The world doesn't get to dictate who you are and what you do, that's for you to own! If you choose, you can be in the driver's seat calling the shots!

You can get, you can be, you can do anything in your life, all you need is confidence. When you dissect your goals, dreams, vision for your life, you'll find that confidence is the way to get to your solutions. It allows you to make moves and call shots in your life that you could never have done otherwise. You get to own the power moves when you have the trust, belief, and security within yourself. You start to look at the world differently. There is nothing you can't do or figure out how to get done. You become limitless. Confidence, like the queen in the game of chess, is the ultimate power player with unlimited moves in this game of life.

Confidence is a mindset. It's a state of being. It's a choice you make. It's comfortable. It's peaceful. It's colorful. It's fun. It's liberating. It's mindful. It's sexy. It's ownership. It's love. It's kindness. It's accepting. It's trust. It's belief. It's faith. It's security. It's like wearing a shoe that fits. You know that no matter what, everything is going to be OK regardless of the outcome. You're ready for everything life throws at you and you welcome new opportunities. Confidence is like doing the tango with the universe. It's passionate, emotional, graceful, it's strikingly beautiful, it's captivating.

I look back at my journey and it makes me sad to think about the woman who didn't want to stand up straight because she thought she was too tall. Makes me sad to think about the woman that didn't value herself and so she accepted anything and everything that came into her life. Makes me sad to think about the girl that believed the comments people told her. If I could go back and talk to my younger self, I would tell her to believe in who she is. Everything she has is enough. Everything she needs is within her. I would tell her to stand firm in who she is because she was made perfect. I would tell her to trust in herself. I would tell her everything is going to be OK. I would tell her that her life is determined by how she chooses to see the world.

My friend, the advice I would give myself is the very definition of confidence and the advice I give to you.

Confidence is queen.

It takes confidence to change your life. It takes confidence to connect with who you are. It takes confidence to be happy. It takes confidence to go after the life you want versus the one you think was handed to you. It takes confidence to stop being a victim. It takes confidence to get in the driver's seat. You are in control if you choose to take control.

Beliefs are the root of your experiences. When you learn you can control your beliefs, thoughts, perceptions, you can turn evil to good and pessimistic to optimistic. You see the world through the lens you want to see. If you choose not to, then your mind will pick for you. The glass may be half full some days and half empty the others. If you don't pick then your mind will flip that coin for you.

If you find yourself in a state of suffering, ask yourself what belief is leading you to feel the way you do. Always be asking yourself if your beliefs and way of thinking serve you. This is the most powerful question you can be asking yourself.

"Whatever the mind can conceive and believe, it can achieve"

-Napoleon Hill

And stop comparing yourself! What do you gain from comparing? You don't know the iceberg under anyone else's story that got them to where they are today. Each one of us is on our own unique journey and no two stories are alike, even your own story with different variables. Comparing is the fastest way to kill or falsely build confidence.

And wherever you are, you're supposed to be right there. Learn to meet yourself where you're at, even if you want to believe you should be further along. Celebrate the small wins and don't wait for the big ones! Life is about the small moments, the small lessons, the baby steps along the way. You'll build your confidence with every step, so don't overlook what may seem small.

Train yourself to be present and look for the gratitude in everything. The joy is in the present, it's the only moment in time we can enjoy. The past is gone and tomorrow isn't guaranteed. Don't miss out on the moments that are happening now. Life is less overwhelming and more enjoyable when you learn the art of being present. How do you eat an elephant? One bite at a time. You'll be more confident when you're not overwhelmed by the unknown of the future.

Connect with your WHY. When you have clarity about purpose then nothing insurmountable gets in your way. Being purpose driven will give you confidence in why you're here, it will give you energy, it will give you the thrust you need to break down any wall in your way. Your purpose is why you're here and the reason to get out of bed in the morning.

And roadblocks, well, they're just opportunities! They help you grow, help you learn, they're the building blocks of your life. Embrace opportunity! When you stop fighting the world then you find your flow. Put energy into your purpose and don't fight your destiny.

You can only control what you can control, don't waste energy on what you can't. When you put energy into what you can't control then you'll find yourself wasting time and moving into suffering. Learn the difference.

You already made the decision that failure is a belief. It's a lesson learned and/or a course correction. You can't fail, so go after an opportunity when it presents itself!

Practice. Practice. Practice! When you practice, you will build that confidence! Get the idea of perfection out of your head and just do the dang thing! Aim for progress over perfection. Perfect is boring anyhow. At all times, give your best, give it your all, operate at 110%, and when you know better-- do better! Practice builds those pathways in your brain to make whatever you're doing second nature, so set your mindset to progress over perfection!

And when you make a decision-- own it. Don't waiver back and forth, be bold about the direction you're taking. If you find that you didn't like the outcome, then take that data and make a different decision next time. Know that whatever you choose is the right course of action for that moment. If you find that it can be done a different way, then do it differently the next time. You're a leader. Leaders pick a direction and go forward. If you need to pivot later- pivot later.

Confidence is positive energy! Be mindful of what energy you allow in your space. The world will always find ways of testing you (just turn on the news), so do what serves you and your energy best.

SET YOUR VALUE!! If you don't set your value then someone else will! Know your worth. Own your kingdom. Don't let anyone come in and devalue you. The only person that should set your value is you and hold everyone else to the value you set. Don't accept less.

Growth will come with discomfort. Just like me getting to 6'1" by the time I was 14 years old, stretching yourself feels weird. But that's your sign that the rainbow is coming. No rainbow comes before the storm. It's natural. It's nature. Grab your rainboots and embrace the feelings.

Even if confidence is an inside job, you can dial it up on the outside too! Confidence isn't made to hide inside, in order to accomplish your goals, you need to actually show up in this world! Don't be afraid to stand out.

Don't be afraid to be different. Don't be afraid to be you unapologetically! That's what makes you special! Put your shoulders back, lock eyes, don't cross your arms, don't fidget, and walk with intention! Put on an outfit you feel good about and do your hair in a way you love! People will see your confidence. People will want what you have. People will love the vibe you put out! And, if they don't, they weren't the right match for you. Do you, queen, do you, and be seen!

Now, my confident queen, I encourage you to always stay humble. There is a huge gap and yet a fine line between confidence and being cocky. Be the person you would want in your own mentor. People will respect and follow someone that has confidence in themself. Being cocky is polarizing and tacky.

Confidence is contagious and people are attracted to confident people. It's a weird phenomenon, but they just do! They'll want to buy your product. They'll want to invest in you. They'll want to be around you. They'll want to get to know you! It all starts from the inside out. Knowing yourself, knowing how to navigate the mind, knowing how to choose your mindset to work for you is going to make you the most powerful player in this game of life.

Trust in yourself. Believe in yourself. Start to say YES more to yourself. Take risks you've never taken. Experience more of what life has to offer. What do you have to lose? Reread this book if excuses are still coming to mind.

Everyone that is breathing is alive, but not everyone that is alive is living. Are you living, or are you existing? When you're 80, will you look back and wish you had or glad you did?

My hope for you is that you look back and know you lived the life you wanted. It's all up to you, you are in control of your mind, if you make that choice.

This is your one shot at this thing we call life. Happen to life, don't let it happen to you. Show life who's boss. Show the world what you have inside of you and allow yourself to be seen. Change the world or just change your world. Whatever you do, I want you to love, trust, and believe in who you are. I want you to have confidence to live your best life, and that a decision that only you can make.

I don't disagree that cash is king, but it won't buy you confidence. Confidence comes from within, and when you have it, you're unstoppable, you're limitless, you're the queen. It's the *way* to your solutions. Practice. Know yourself. Love yourself. Thank yourself. Embrace your unique gifts. And know that you are right where you are supposed to be. Celebrate. Enjoy the journey. Create the life you want to lead, one thought at a time.

Confidence is everything. Confidence is what makes that simple white tee and jeans look good.

-Ciara

ABOUT THE AUTHOR

Jen Sugermeyer lives in Dallas, Texas with her cat, Booger. Since everything is bigger in Texas, Jen knew she'd be a good fit being 6'1"!

After a successful corporate career as a leader in IT, Jen left to pursue her purpose of helping others take control of their lives and their businesses through coaching and speaking.

Jen loves bringing her energy, her stories, and her heels to motivate and transform lives.

Are you happening to life-
Or is life happening to you?

You can find her services, morning mindset show, podcast, socials, and more at:

www.jensugermeyer.com